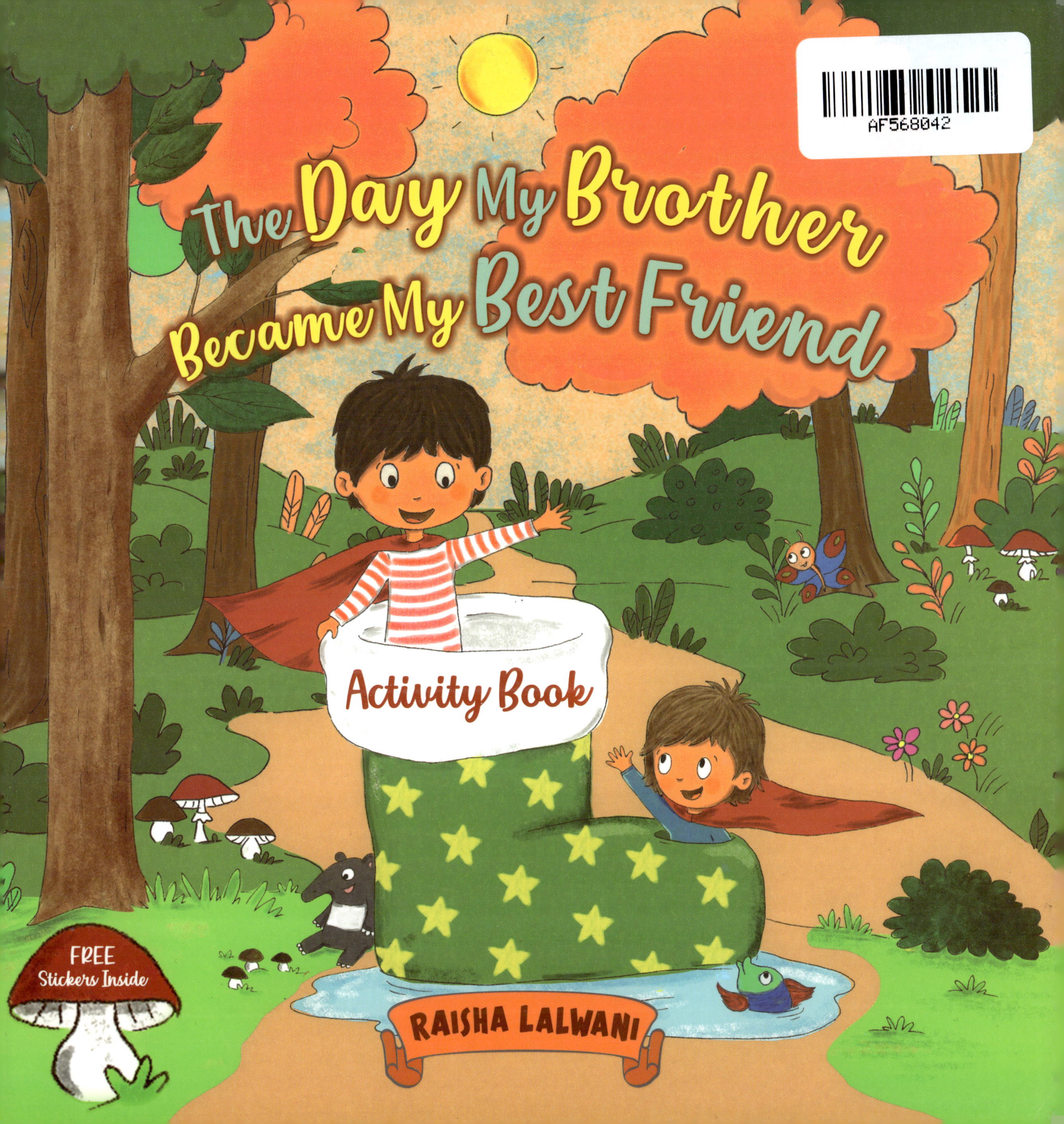
AF568042
The Day My Brother Became My Best Friend
Activity Book
RAISHA LALWANI
FREE
Stickers Inside

The Day My Brother Became My Best Friend

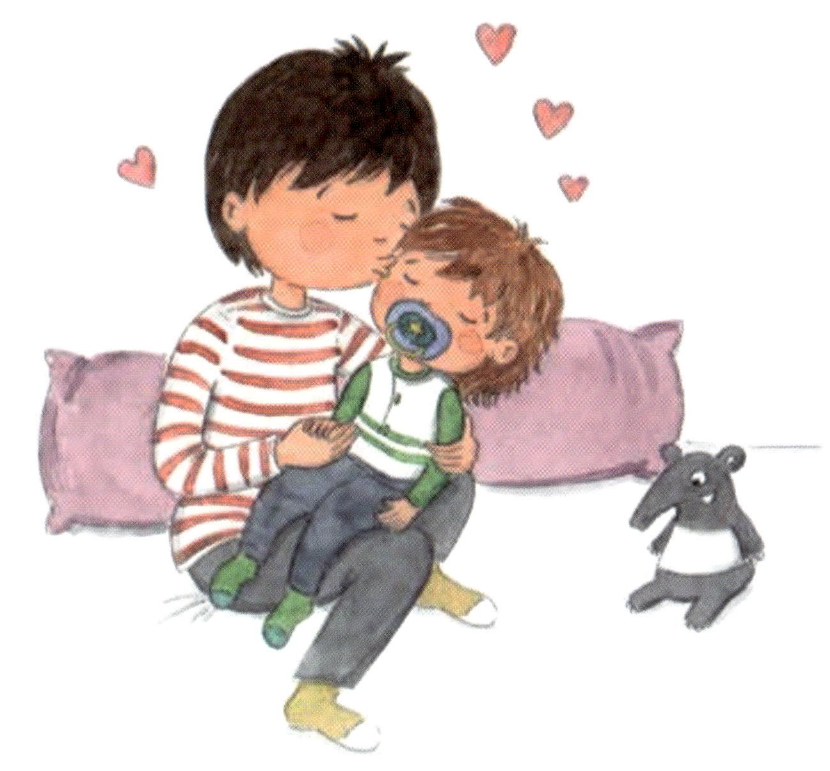

Activity Book

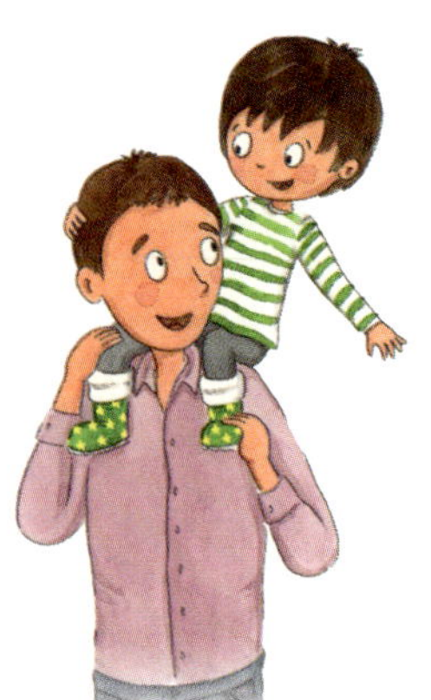

Word Search

Let's help Ben find the Names of his Family Members

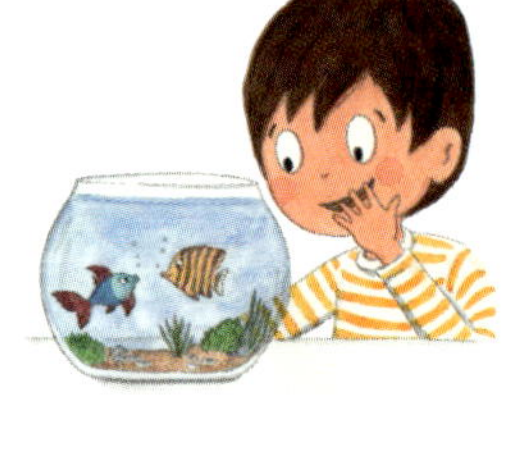

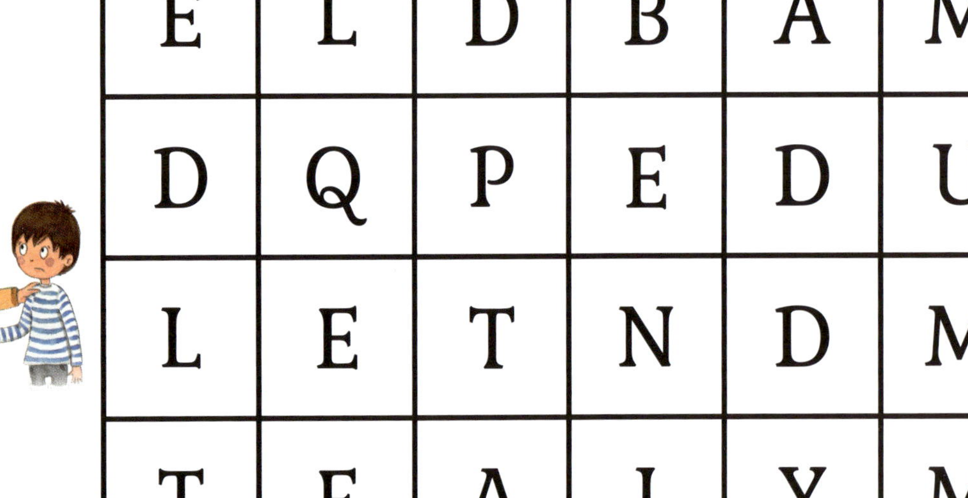

G	R	A	N	D	P	A
E	L	D	B	A	M	N
D	Q	P	E	D	U	D
L	E	T	N	D	M	R
T	F	A	I	Y	M	E
P	R	B	O	X	Y	W
G	K	X	N	P	F	X

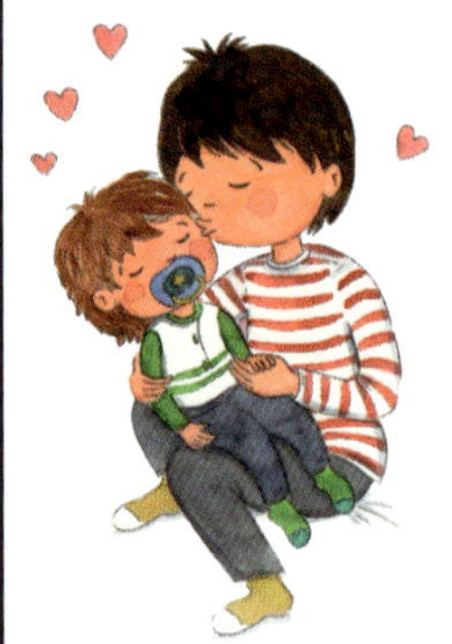

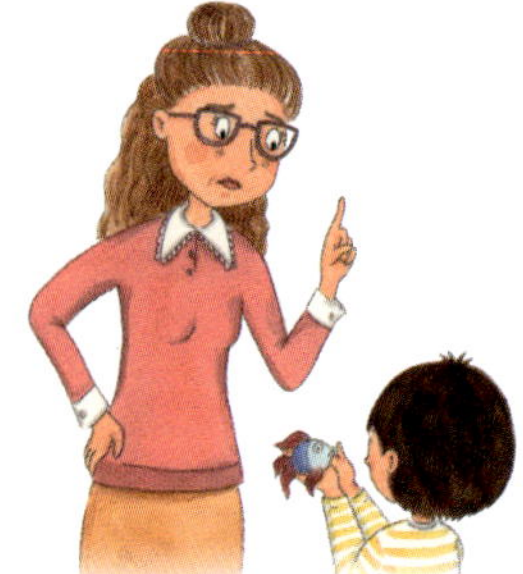

Ben	Andrew	Daddy
Mummy	Grandpa	Grandma

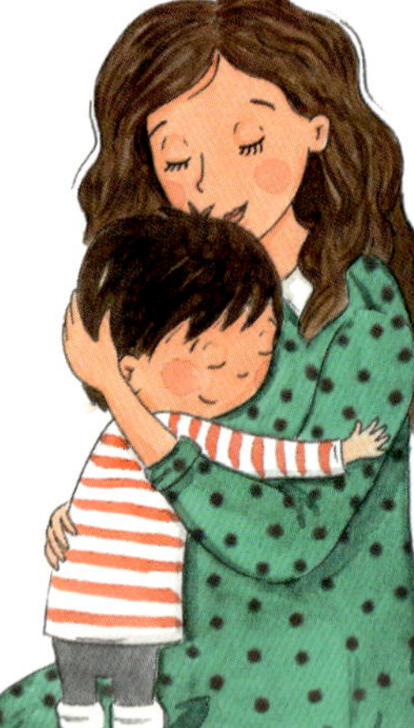

Family

Concern — Love — Care — Understanding — Unity

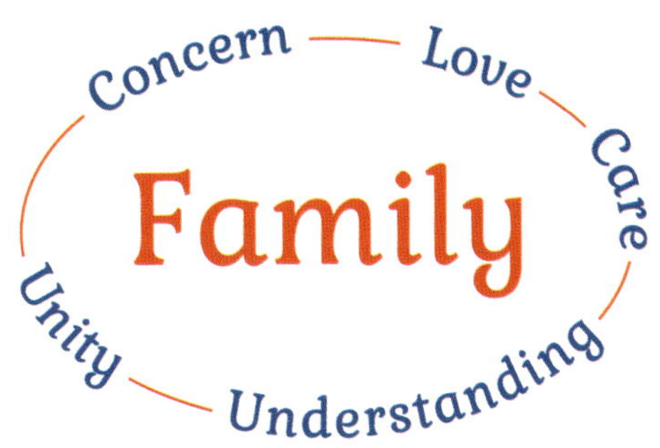

Task 1: Paste a Family Picture.

Task 2: Design Your own Frame (You may use Straws/Buttons/Stickers/Colours).

Task 3 (Optional): Cut the Frame and Paste it in your Room.

Spot the Difference

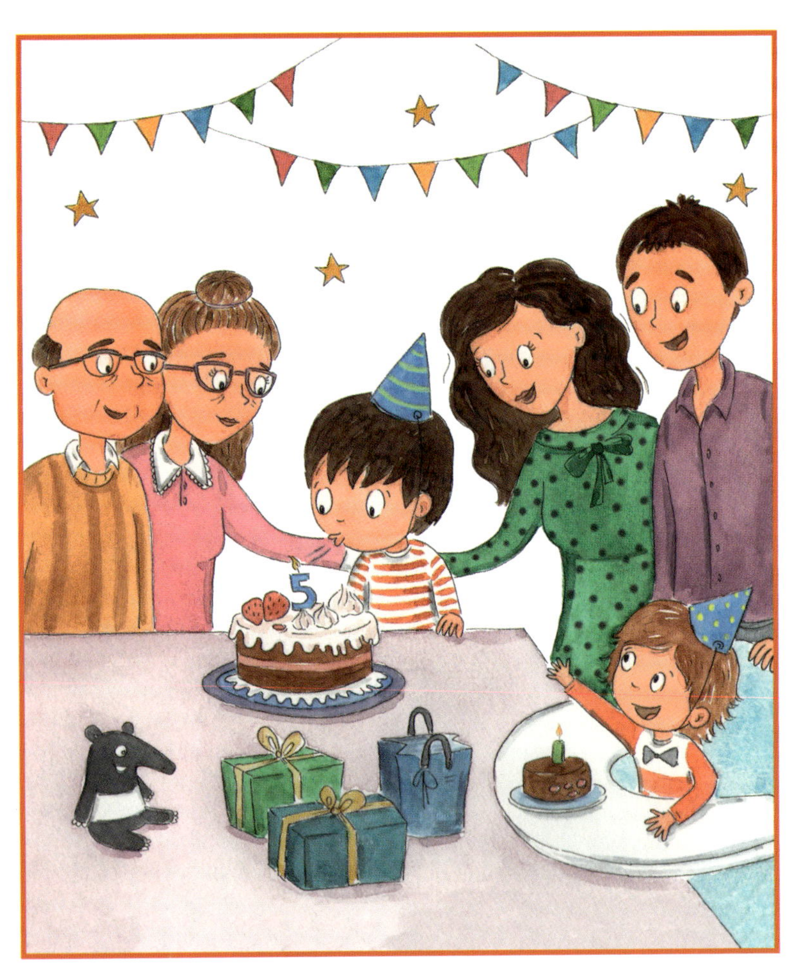

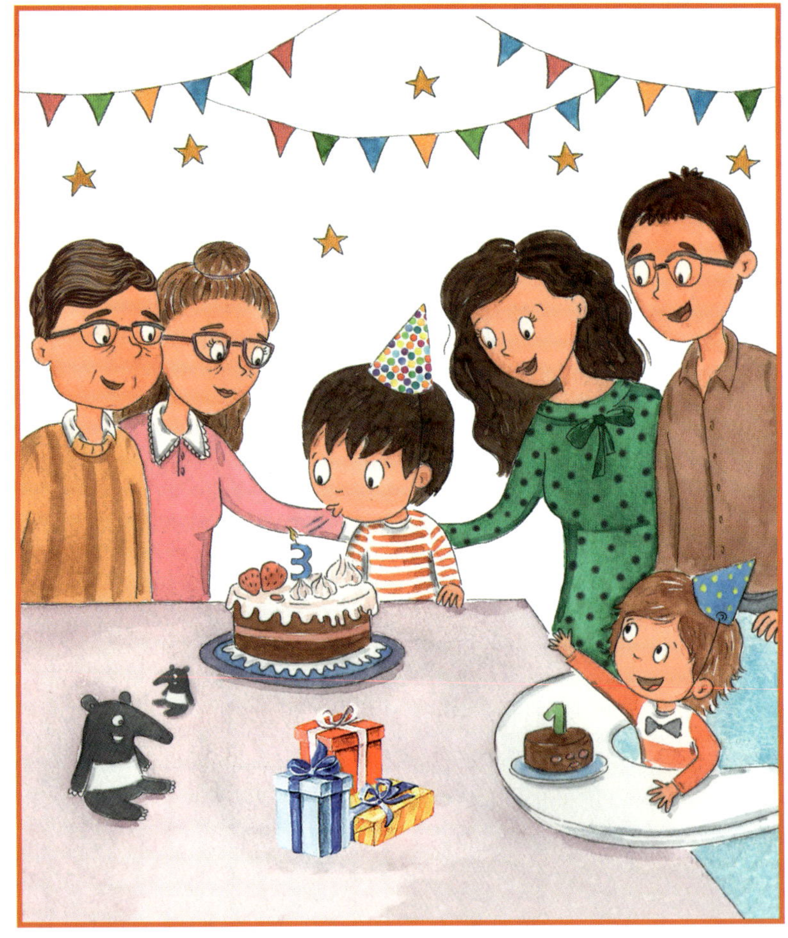

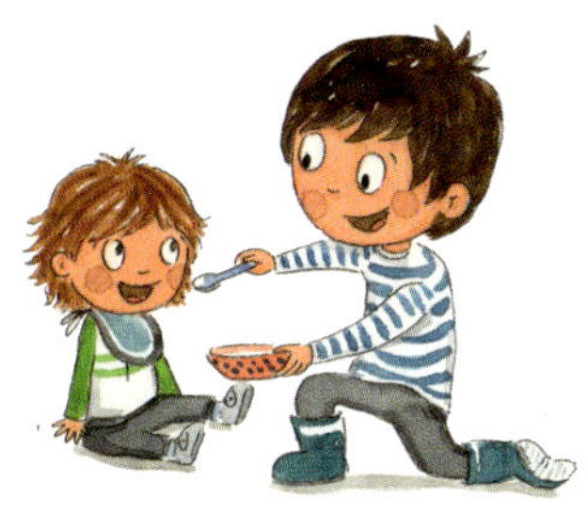

Make a list of all the fun things you would like to try with your brother / sister / friend:

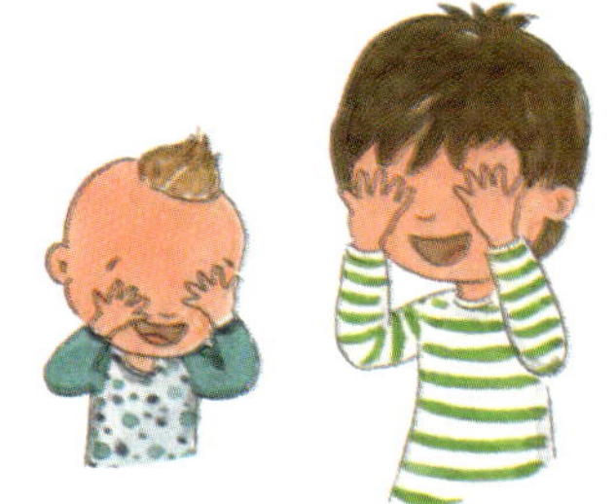

1. Make up a code language that only we can understand.

2. ....

3. ....

4. ....

5. ....

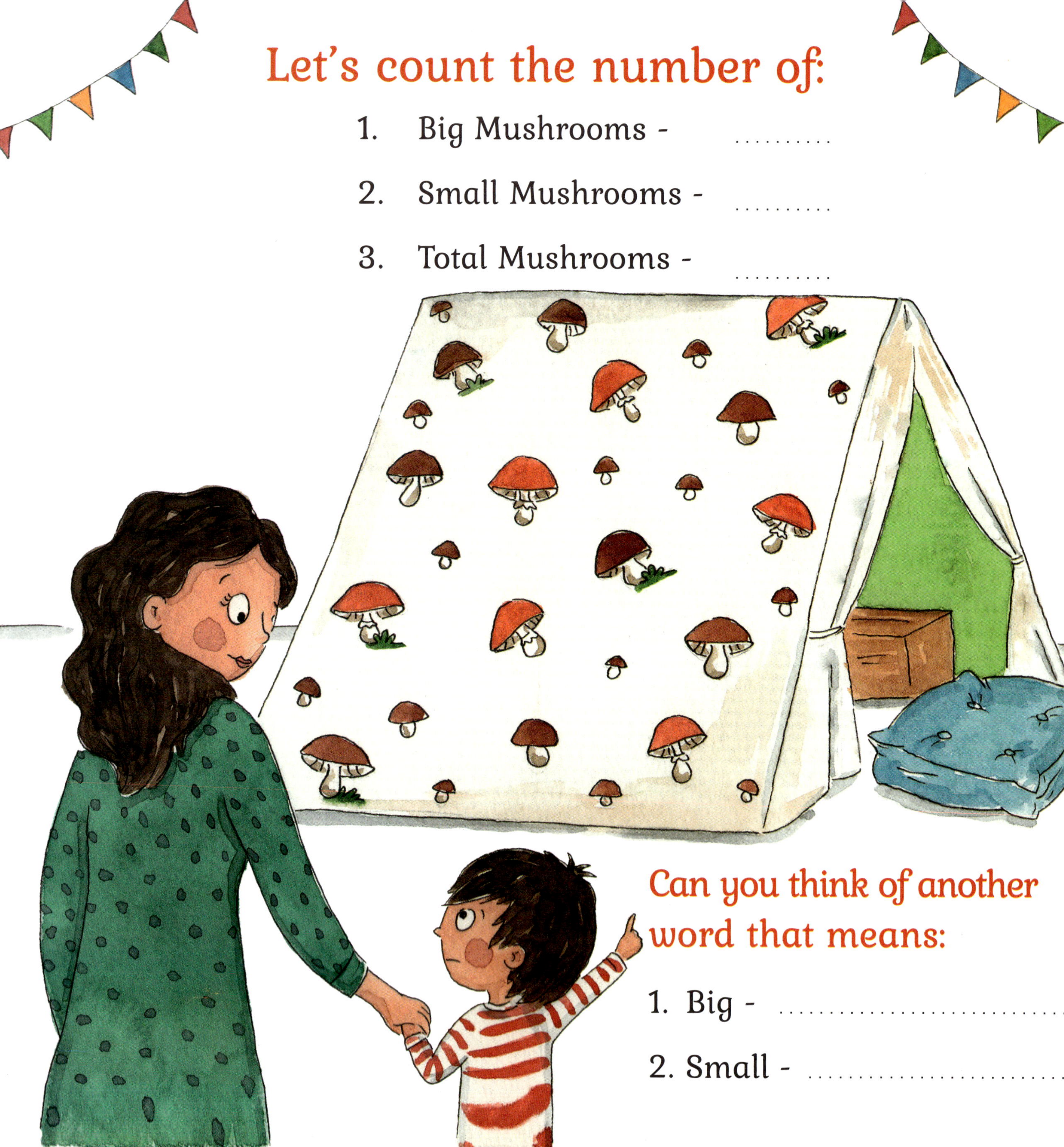

Let's count the number of:

1. Big Mushrooms - ....
2. Small Mushrooms - ....
3. Total Mushrooms - ....

Can you think of another word that means:

1. Big - ....
2. Small - ....

Connect the Dots

Let's Draw and Colour Ben's Favourite Toy 'Tapir'

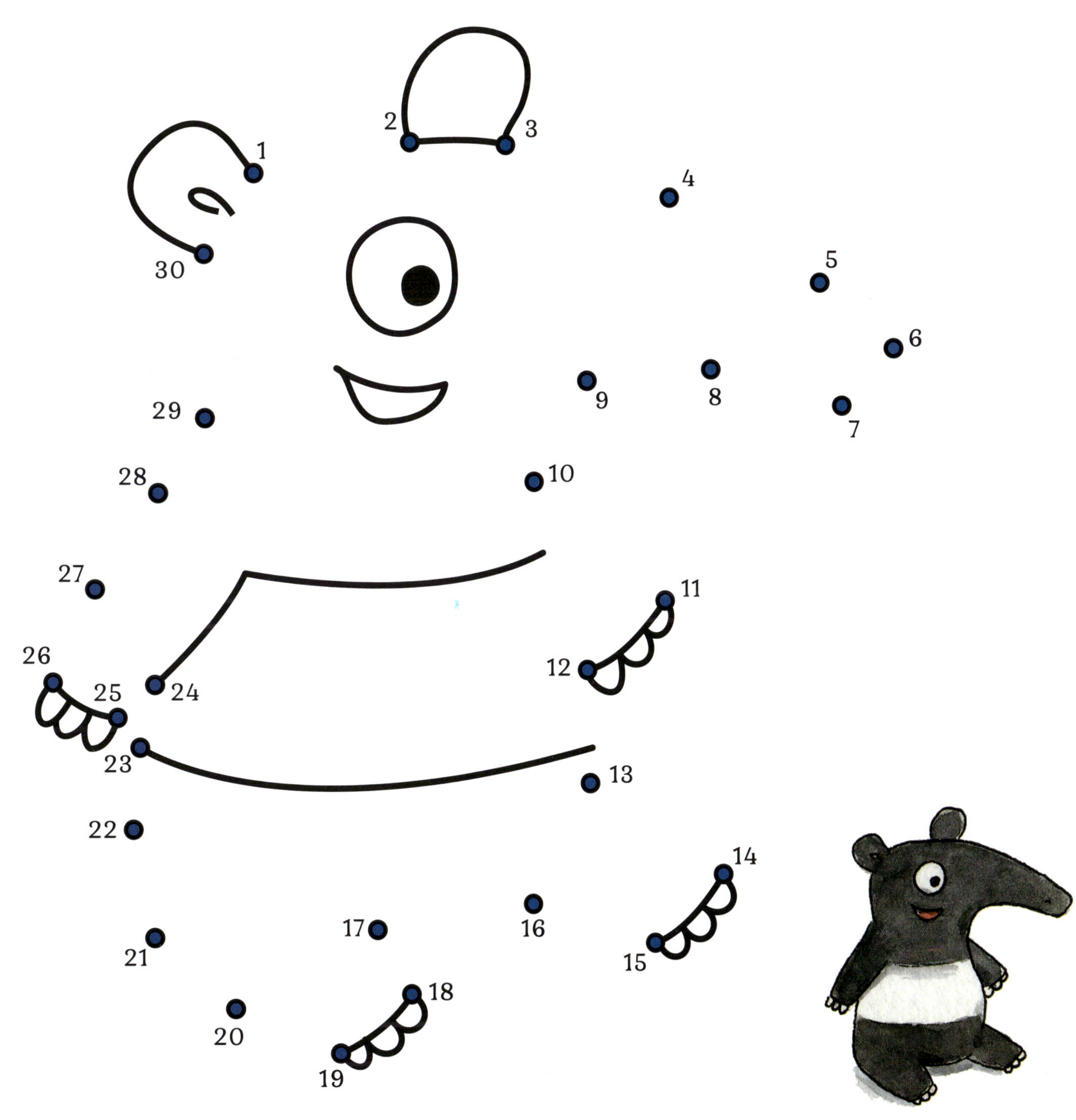

When we talk about the things that we / someone is doing right now, we use:

Person + is / am / are + Action Word + *ing* + ...

Example: Ben is hugging his Mummy.

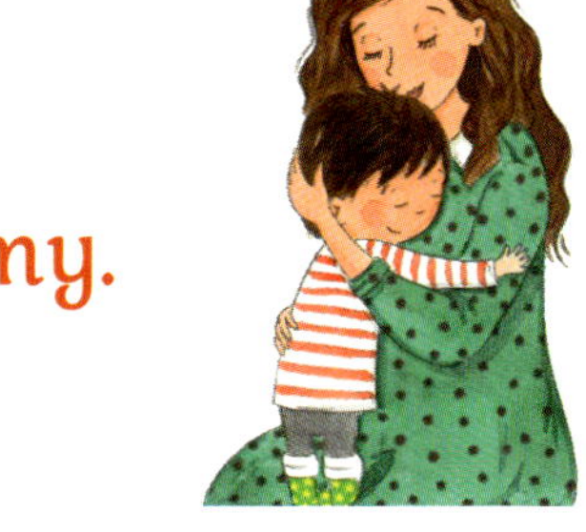

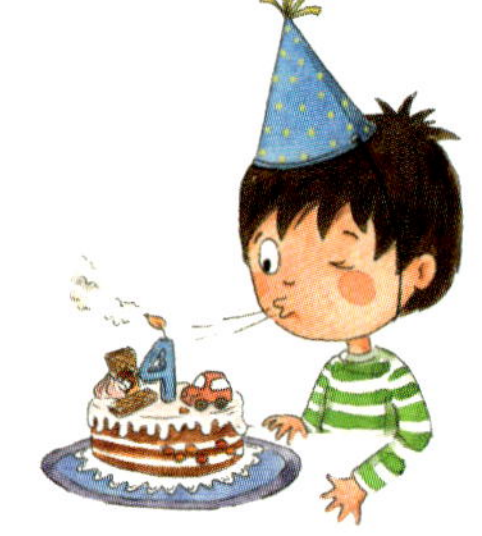

1. Ben .... his birthday candle. (blow)

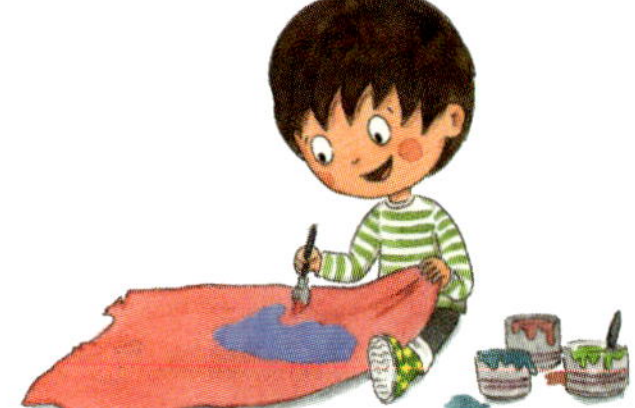

2. Ben .... his cape. (paint)

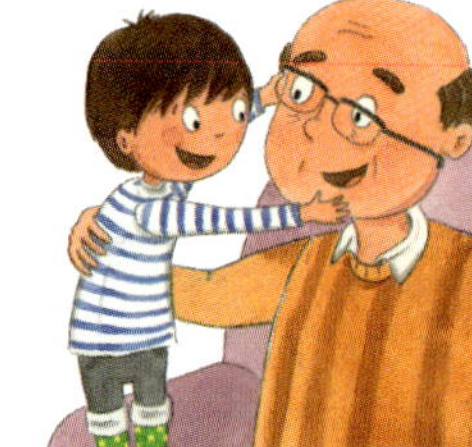

3. Ben .... with his Grandpa's glasses. (play)

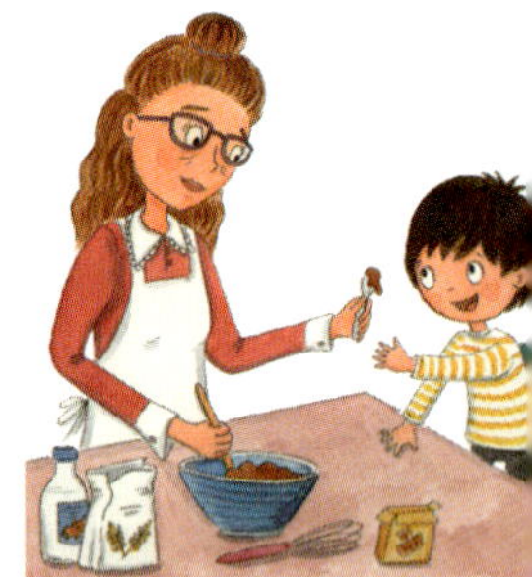

4. Ben .... his Grandma bake a cake. (help)

Ben to Andrew's Rescue

Let's help Ben find his way
to his little brother Andrew

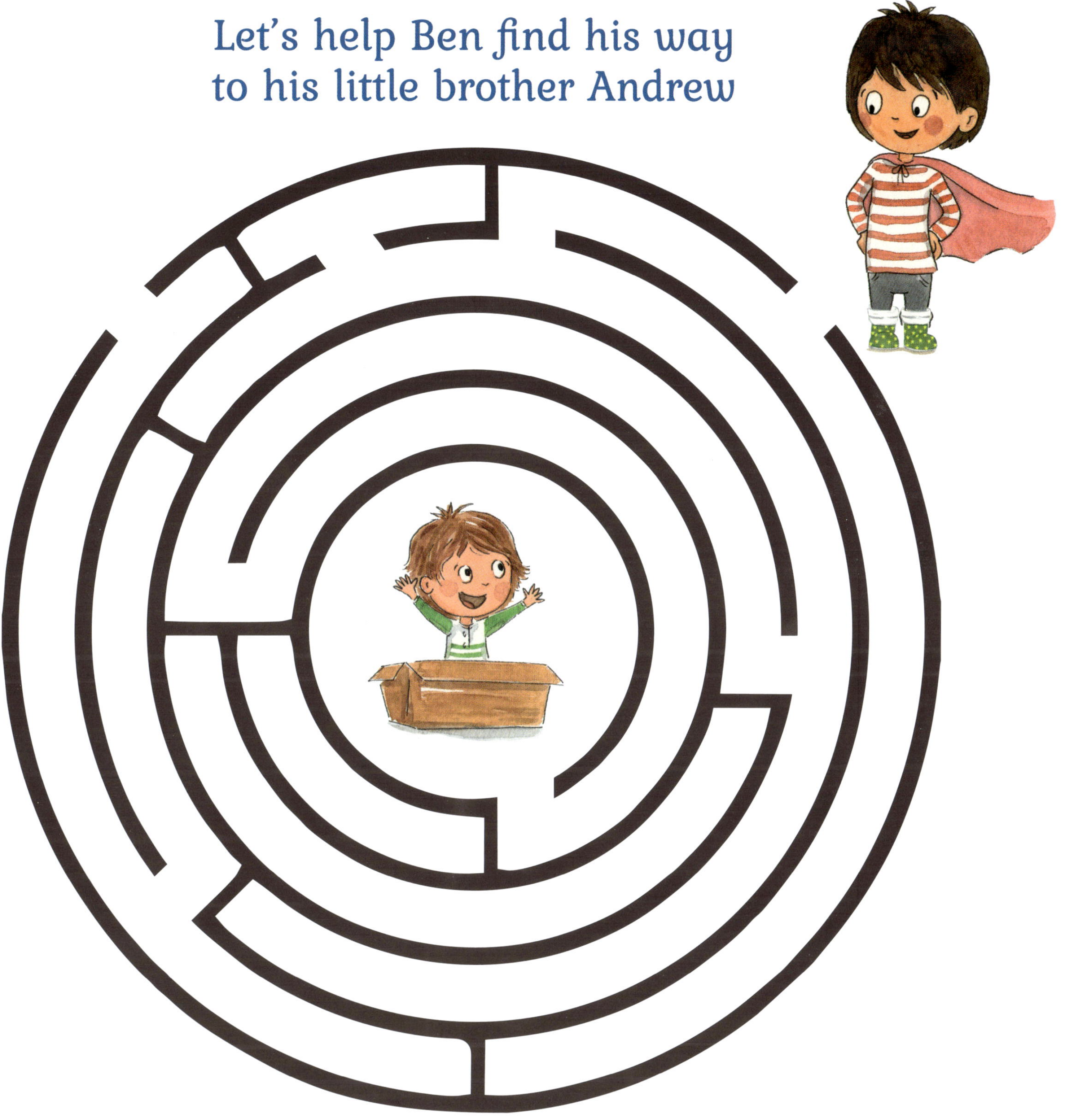

Let's Design

Ben has out-grown his shoes.
Let's design a new pair for him.

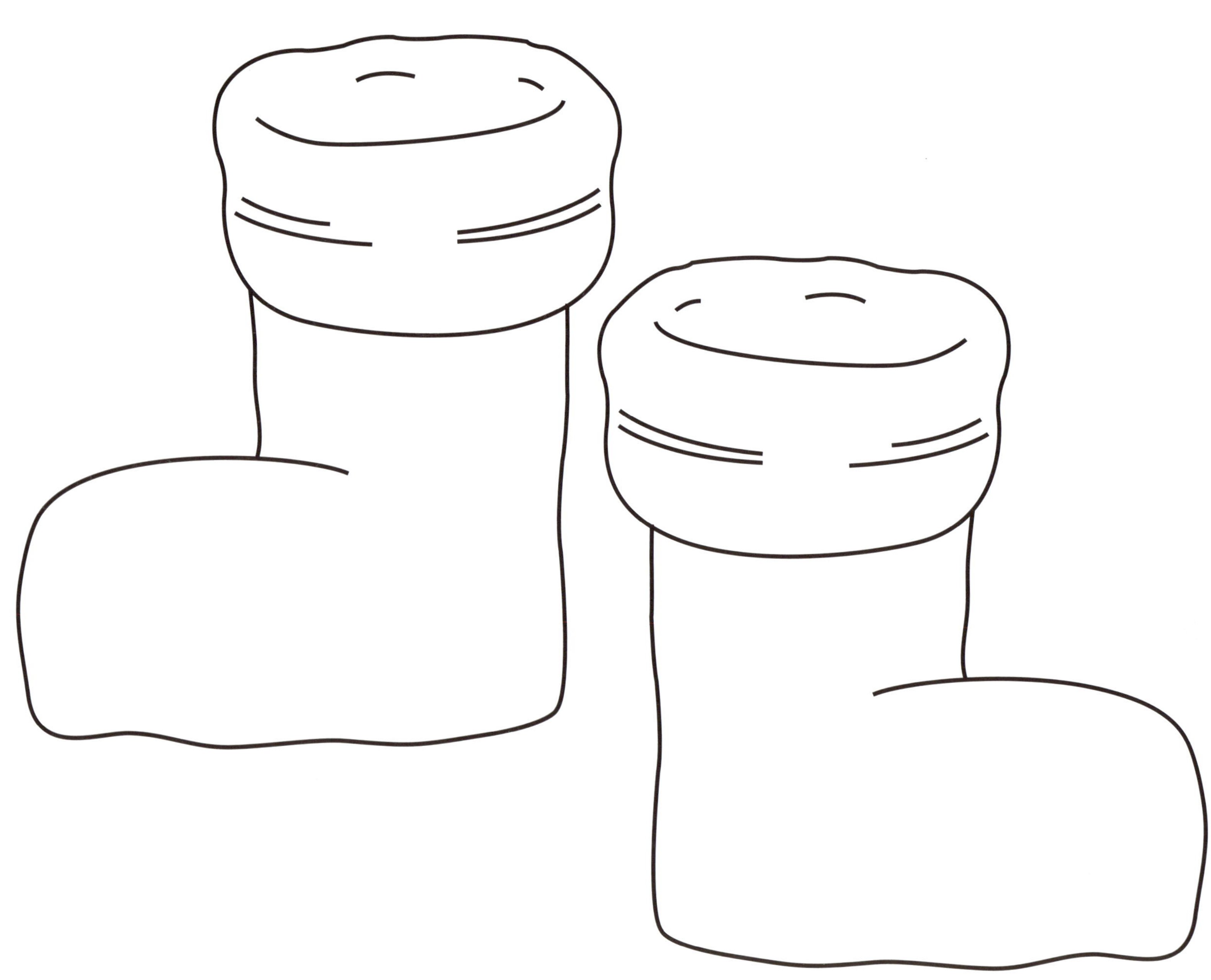

Let's be Creative

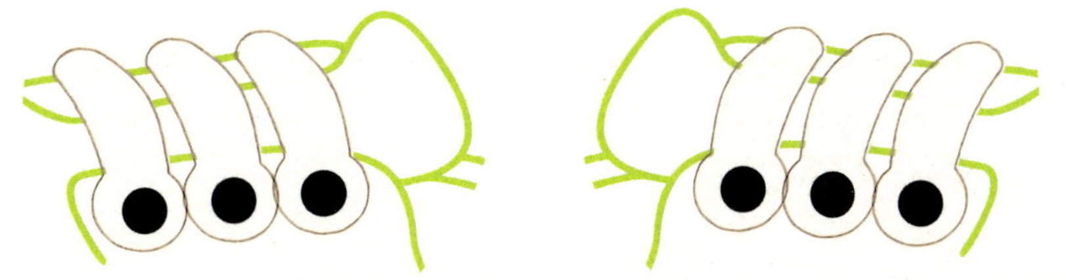

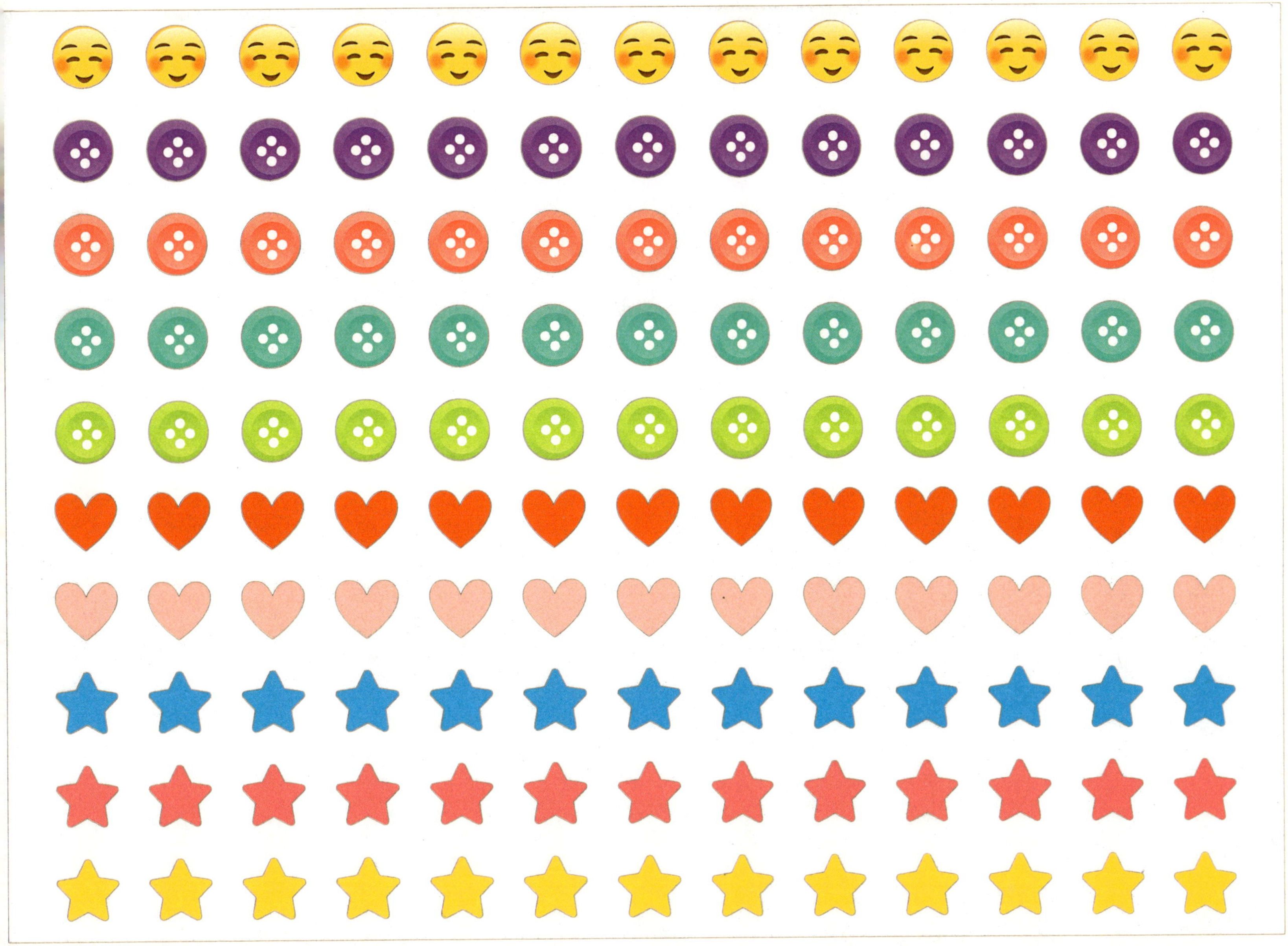

Let's be Creative

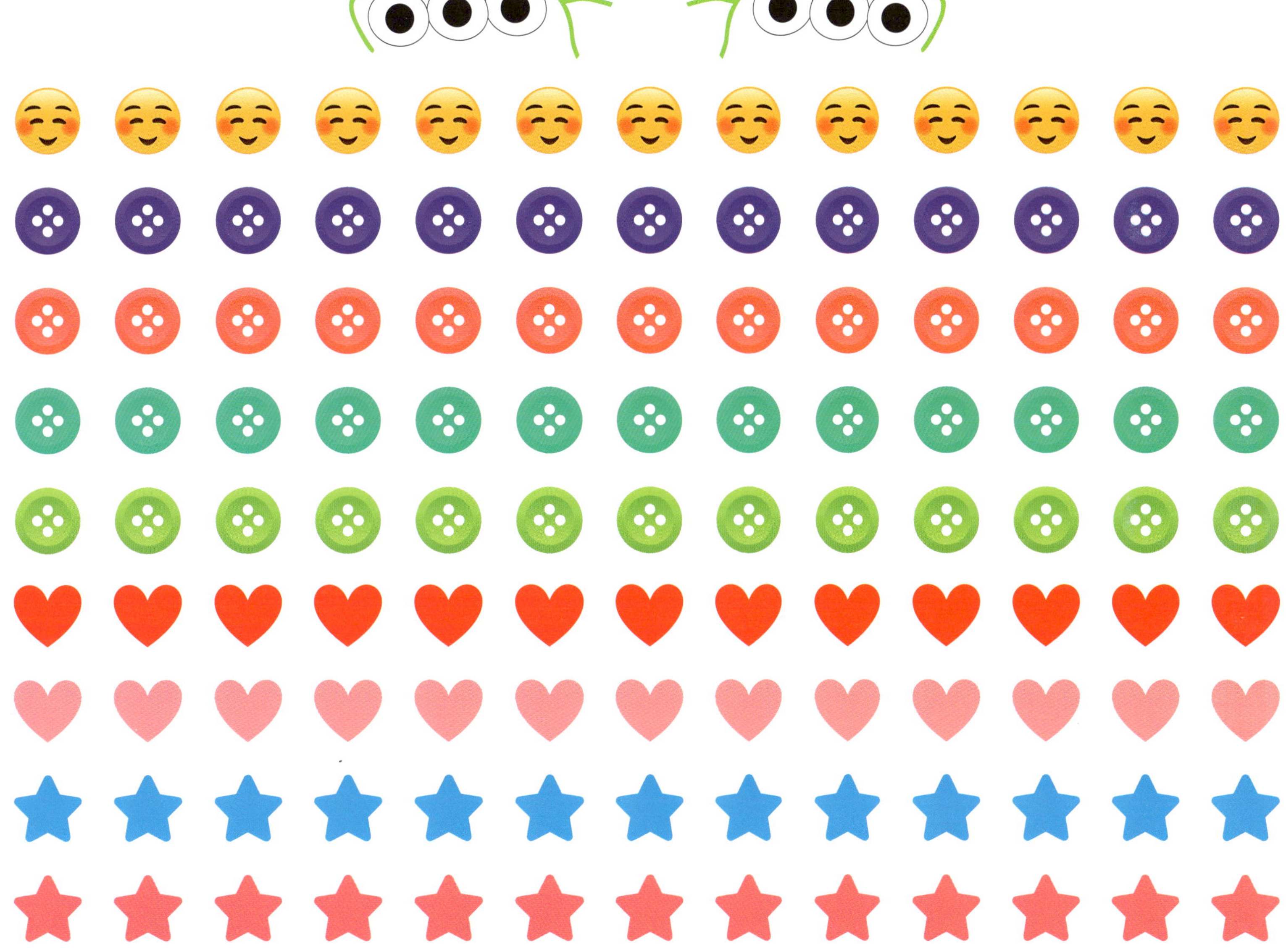

1. When is your Birthday ?

My Birthday is on ________________

2. How old will you turn on your upcoming Birthday ?

I will turn ______________________

3. Which flavour of cake would you like ?

I would like a/an ___________________________

___________________________ for my Birthday.

4. Design your future Birthday Cake.

5. Draw the number of candles on your cake.

6. Make a Birthday Wish.

(Be Realistic)

____

____

____

____

____

____

____

____

Cake Time

The Day My Brother Became My Best Friend

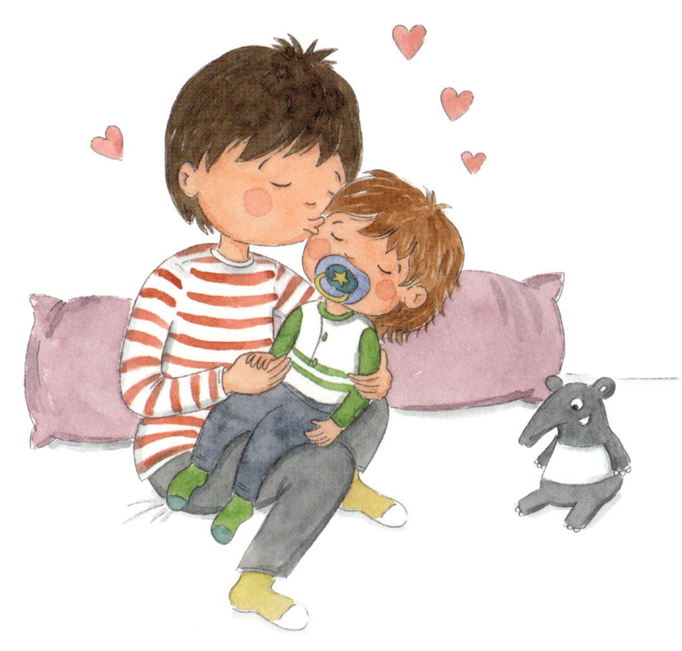

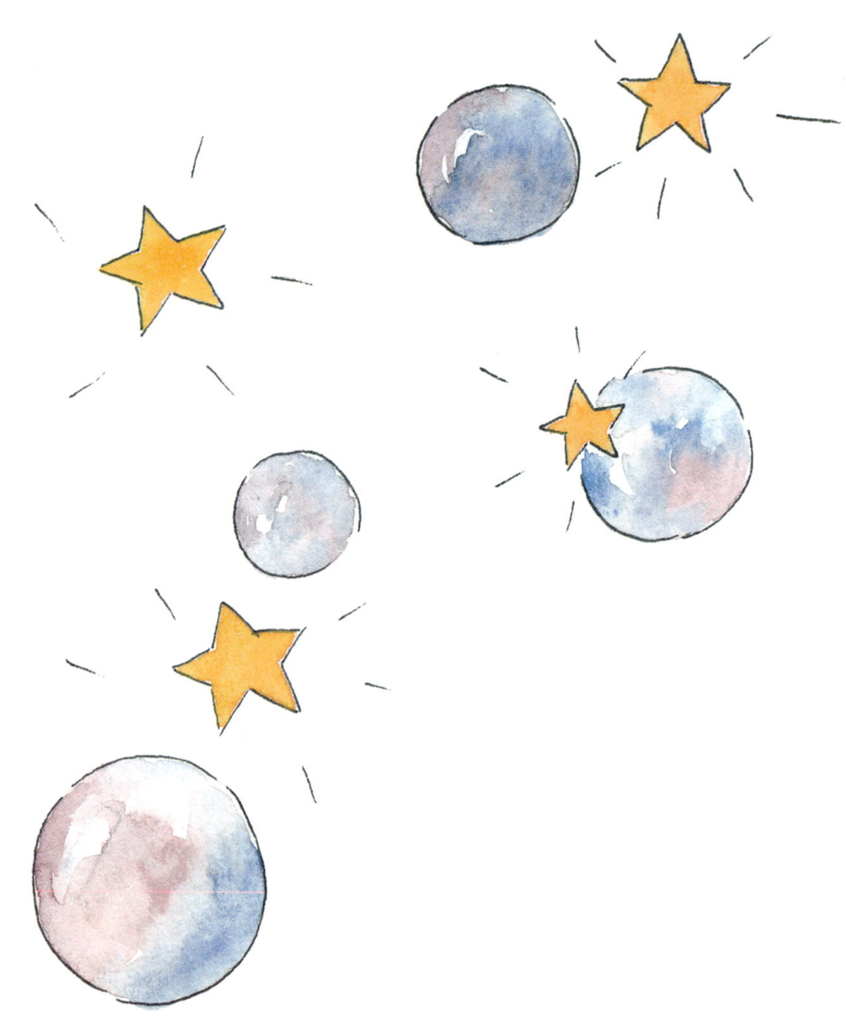

The Day My Brother Became My Best Friend

RAISHA LALWANI

Illustrated by
Dagmar Chládková

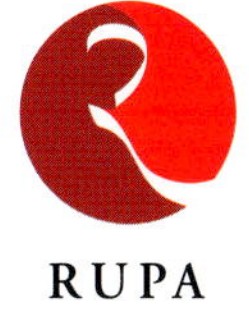

RUPA

Published by
Rupa Publications India Pvt. Ltd 2021
7/16, Ansari Road, Daryaganj
New Delhi 110002

Sales centres:
Allahabad Bengaluru Chennai
Hyderabad Jaipur Kathmandu
Kolkata Mumbai

ISBN: 978-93-91256-00-5

First impression 2021

10 9 8 7 6 5 4 3 2 1

Printed at Thomson Press India Ltd., Faridabad

For my heartbeats,
Abhiraj and Rajveer

May your life be filled
with beautiful stories

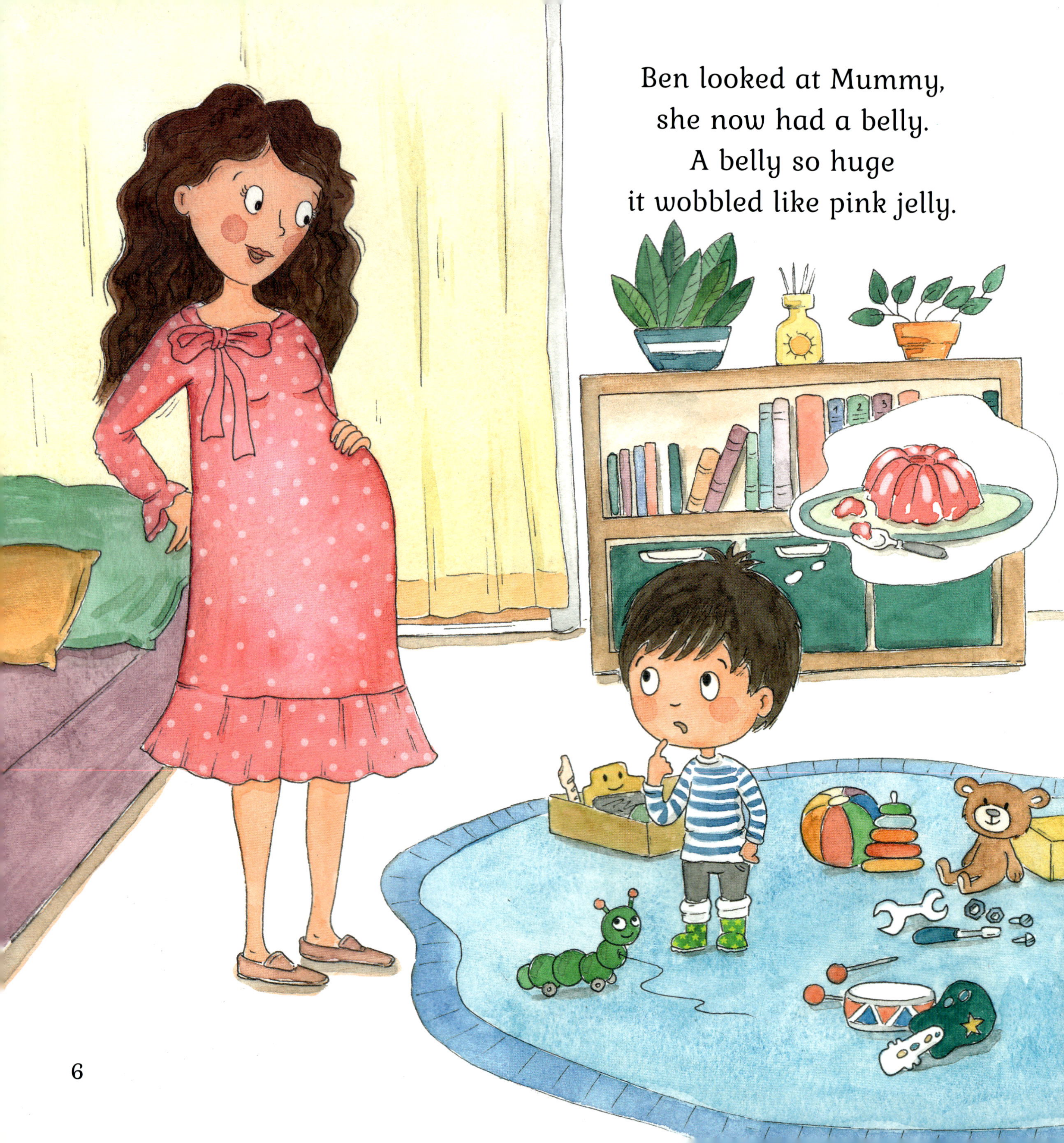

Ben looked at Mummy,
she now had a belly.
A belly so huge
it wobbled like pink jelly.

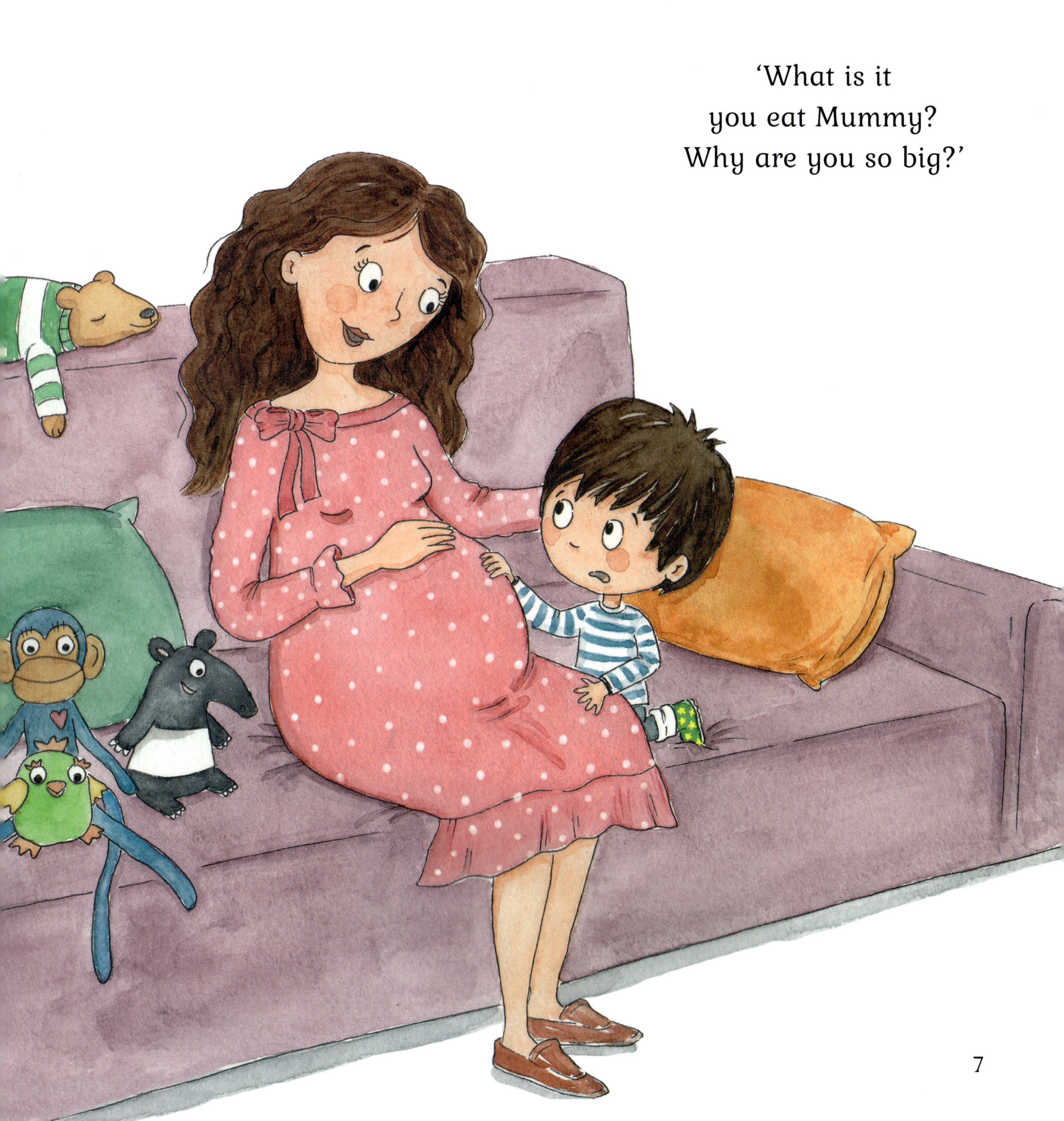

‘What is it
you eat Mummy?
Why are you so big?’

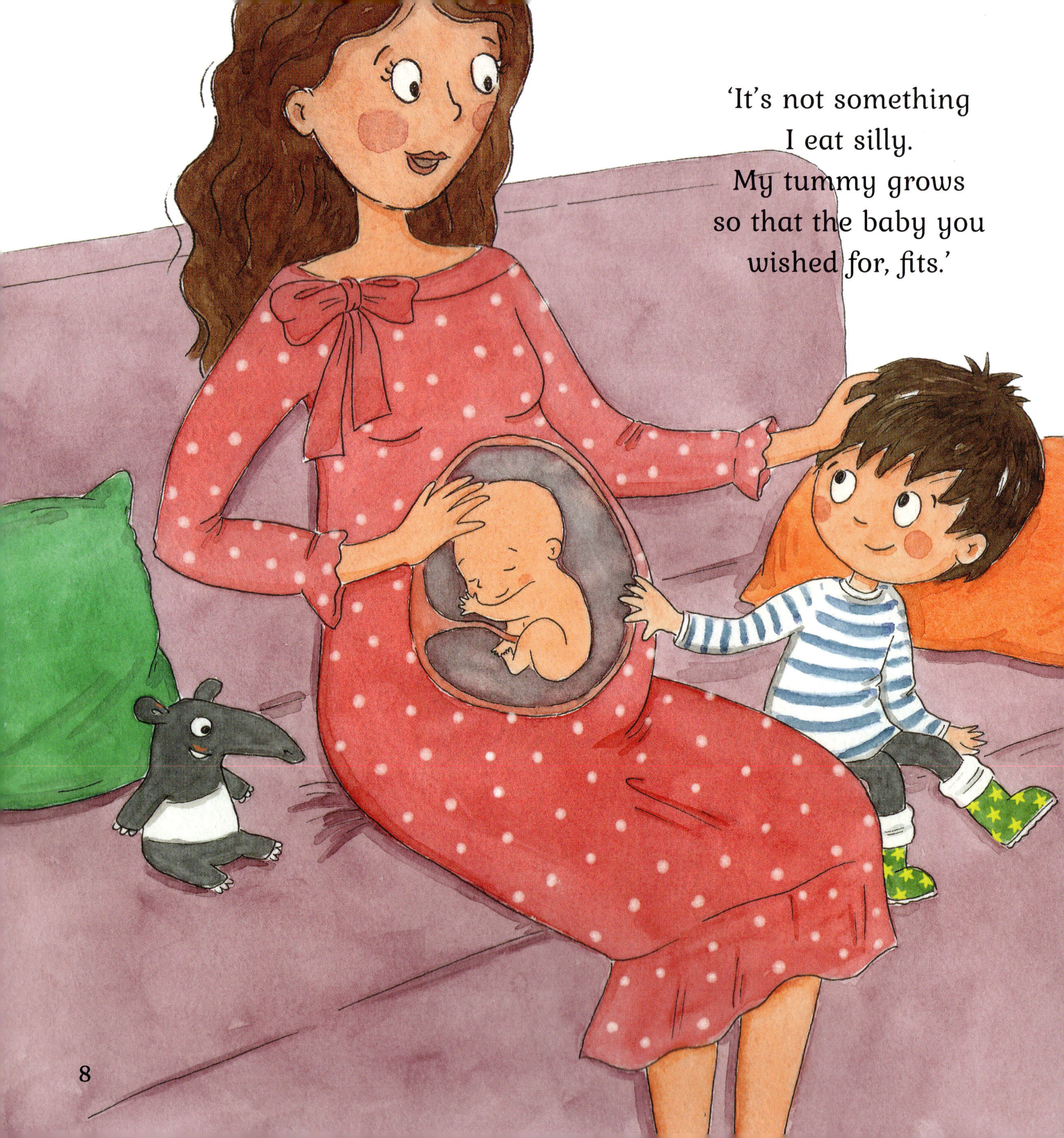

'It's not something
I eat silly.
My tummy grows
so that the baby you
wished for, fits.'

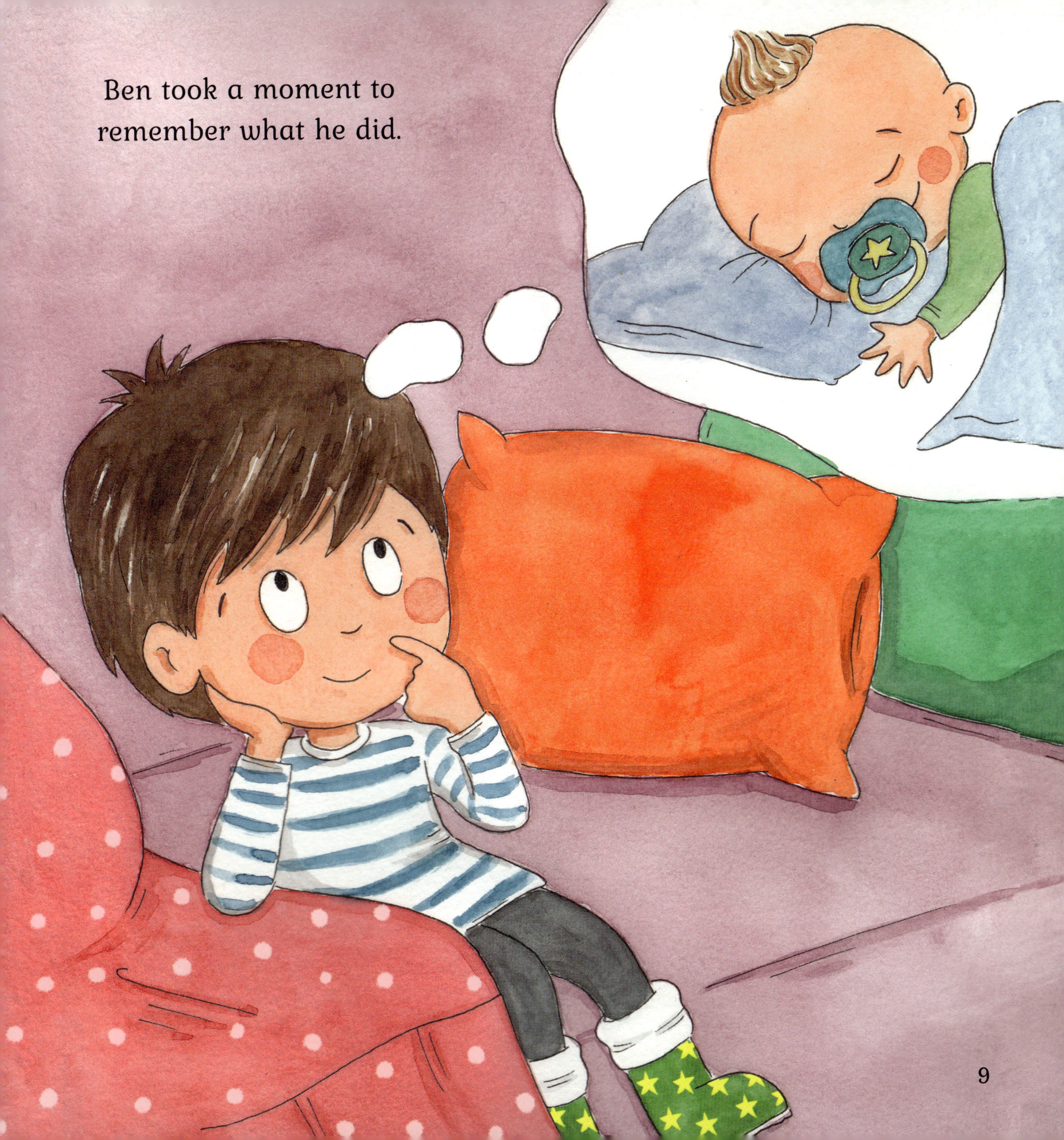

Ben took a moment to
remember what he did.

He had asked for a baby,
As his fourth birthday wish.

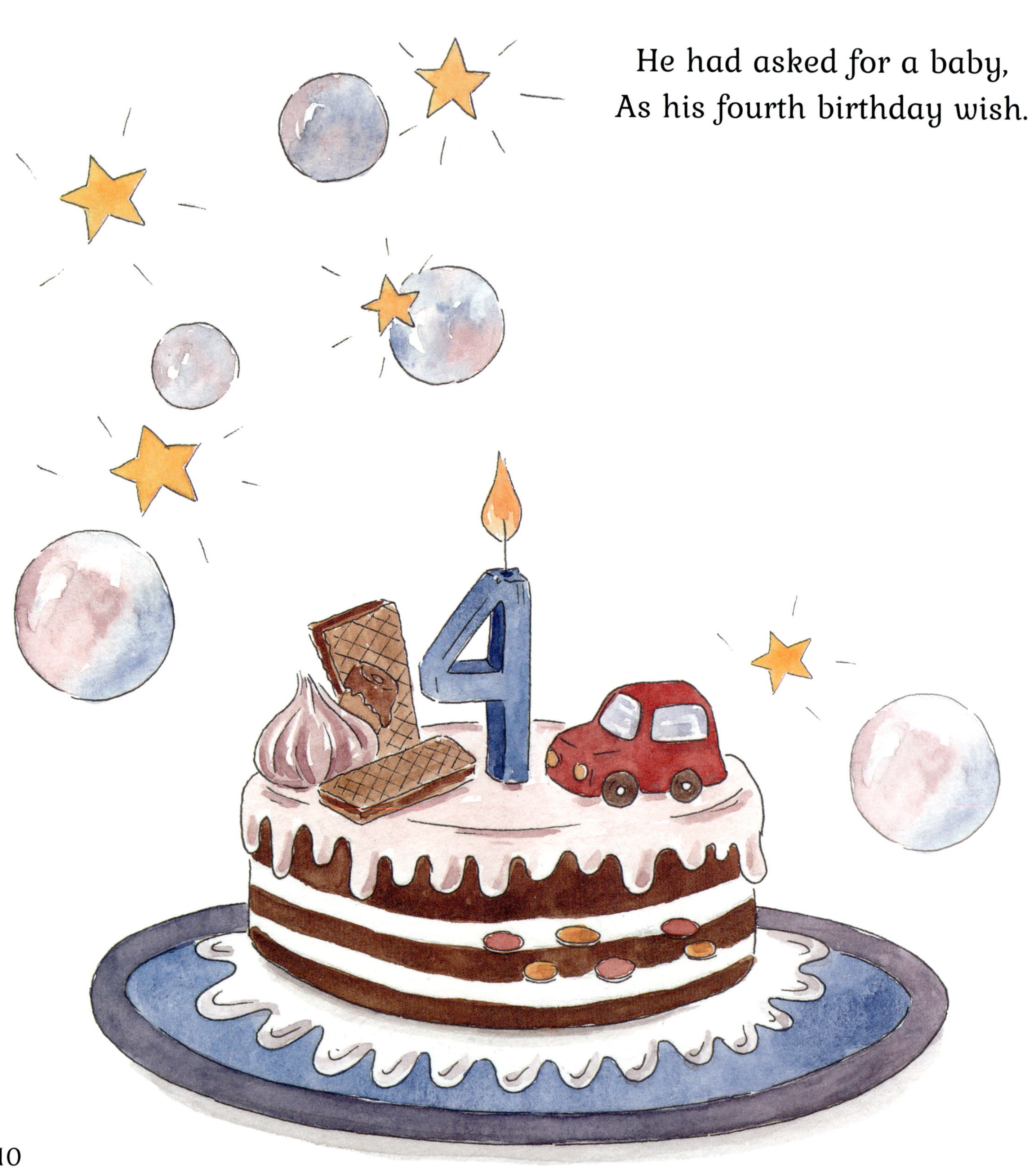

So few weeks later,
when Santa dropped by,
he must've cleaned the chimney
because along with all the
presents,
a baby came by.

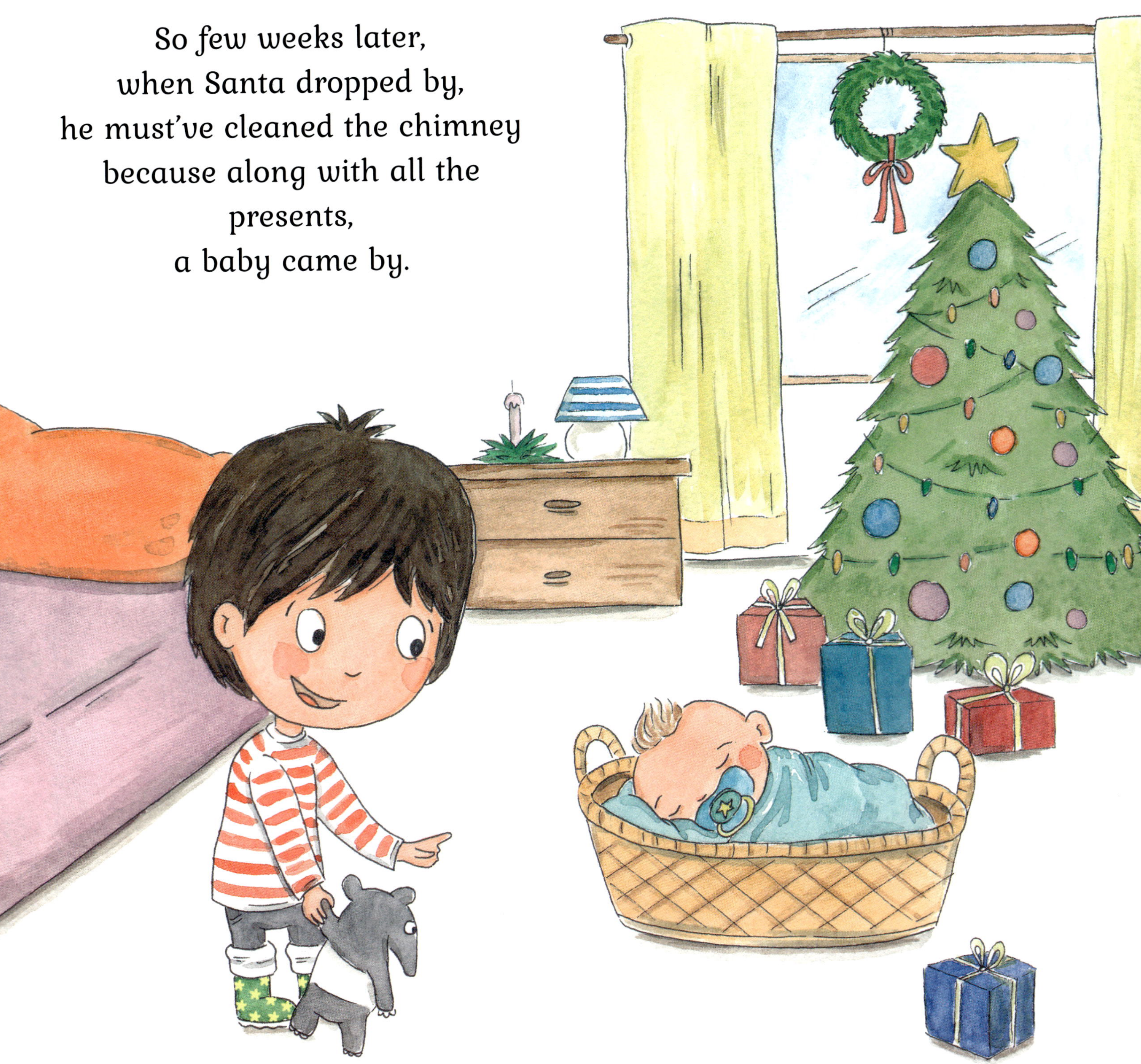

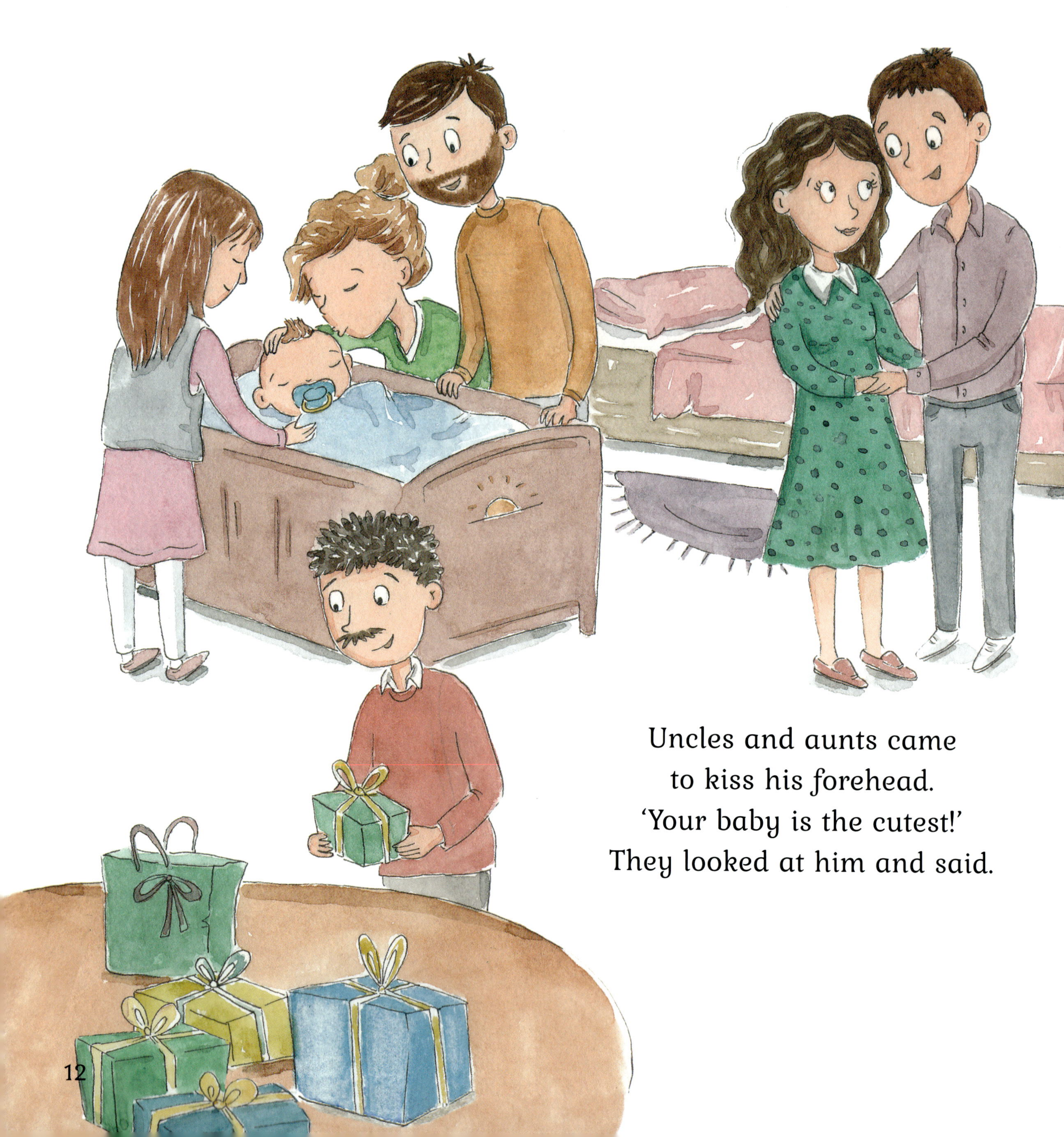

Uncles and aunts came
to kiss his forehead.
'Your baby is the cutest!'
They looked at him and said.

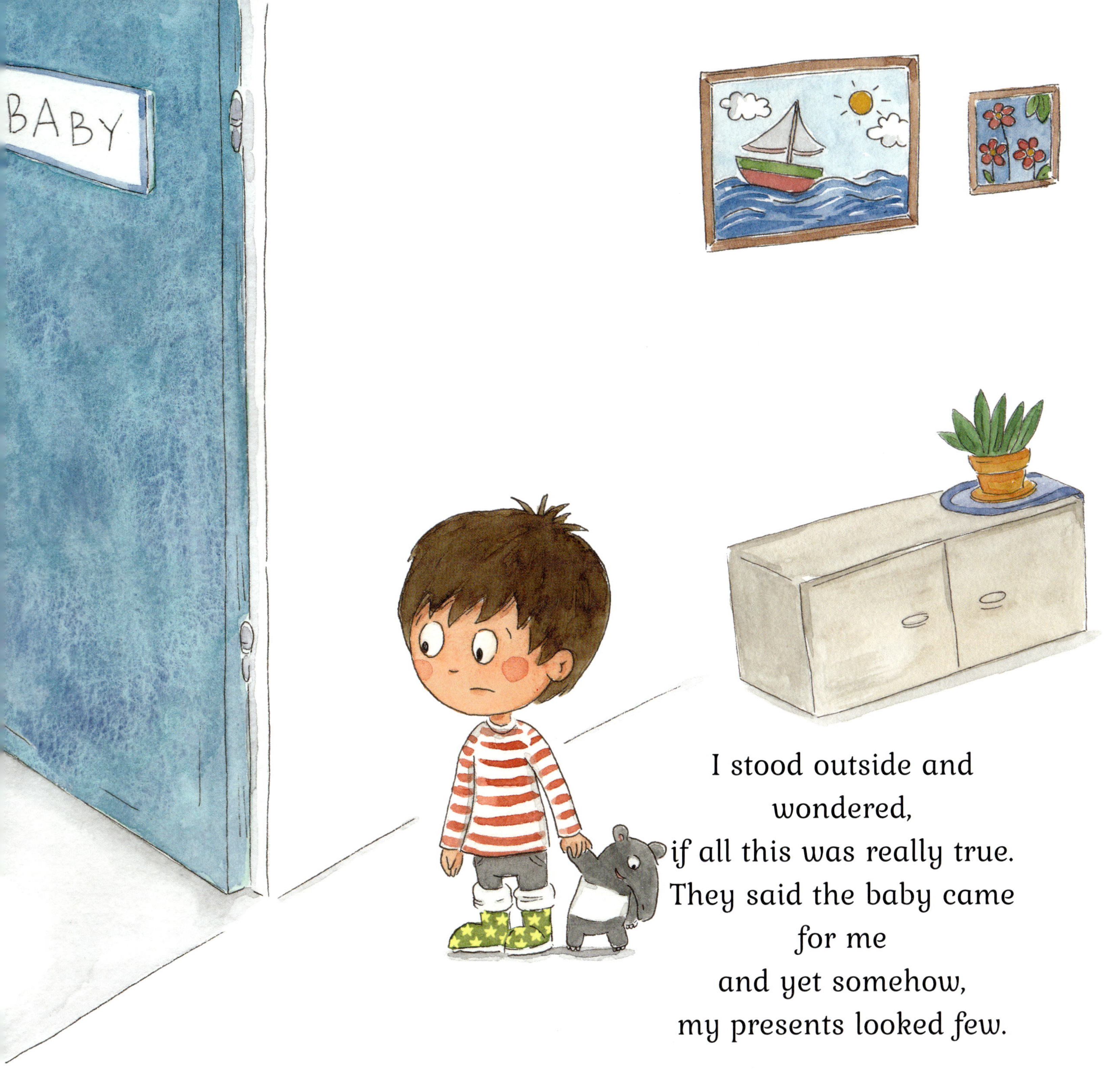

I stood outside and
wondered,
if all this was really true.
They said the baby came
for me
and yet somehow,
my presents looked few.

I turned around
began to walk
to find old toys and play

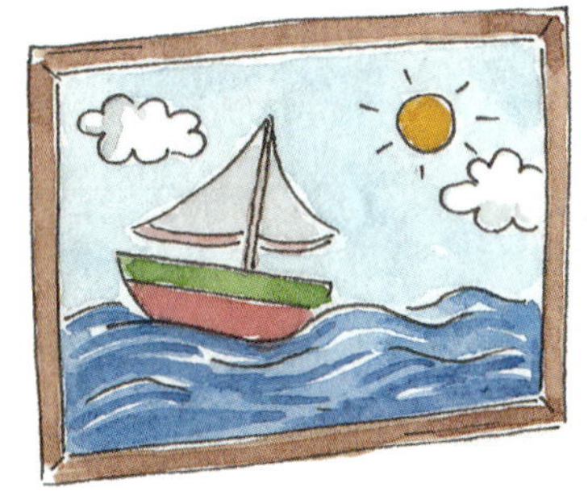

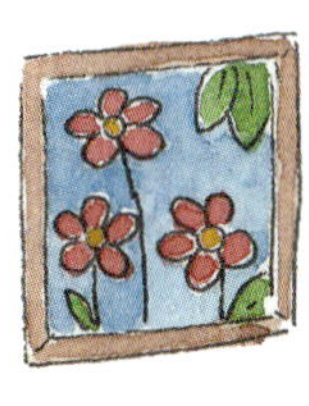

When Mummy came and hugged me.
She told me 'Don't move!
For a moment, just stay.'

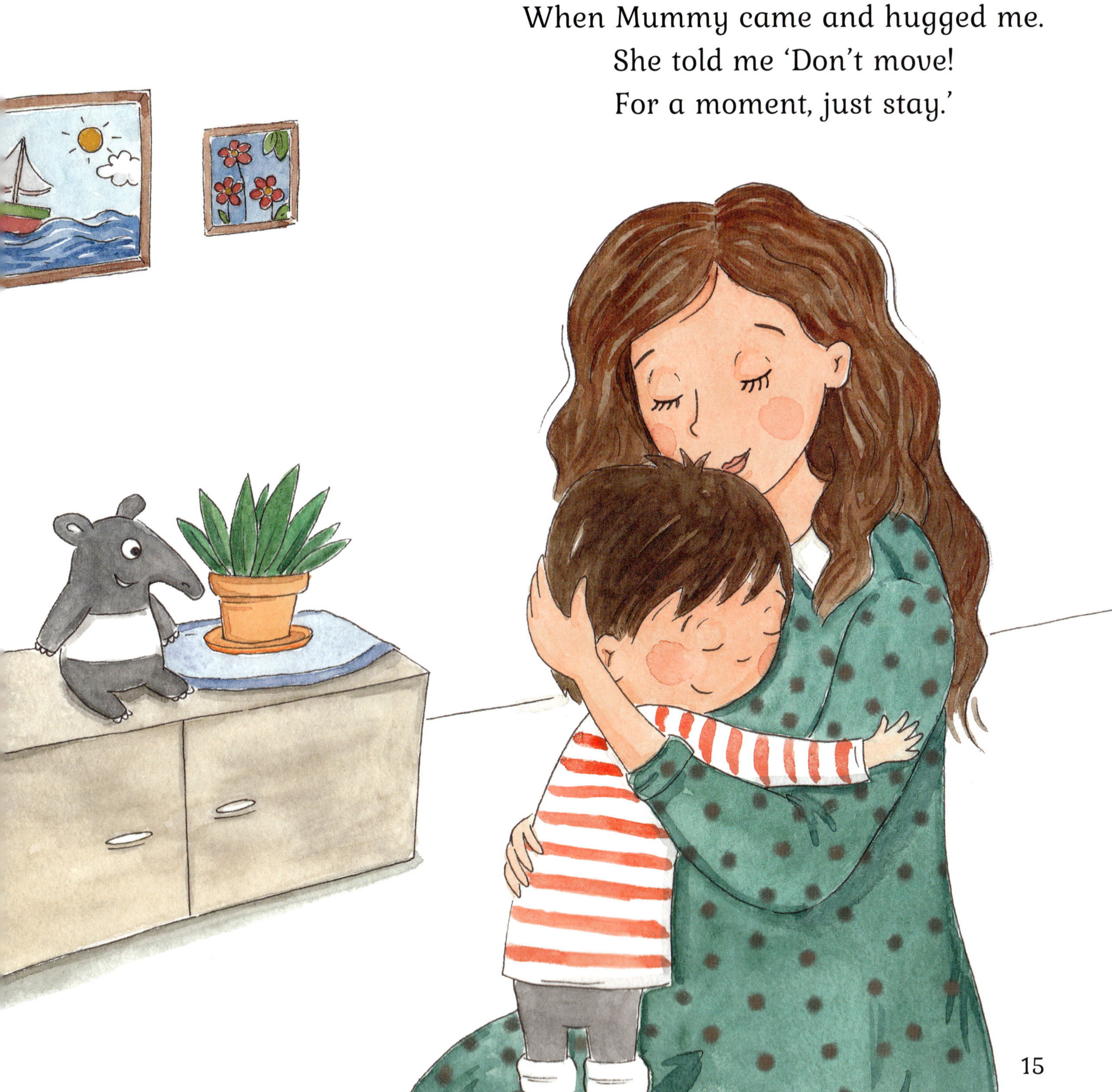

She held me by my hand
and then took me to my room
where I saw a camping tent
that looked a lot like mushrooms.

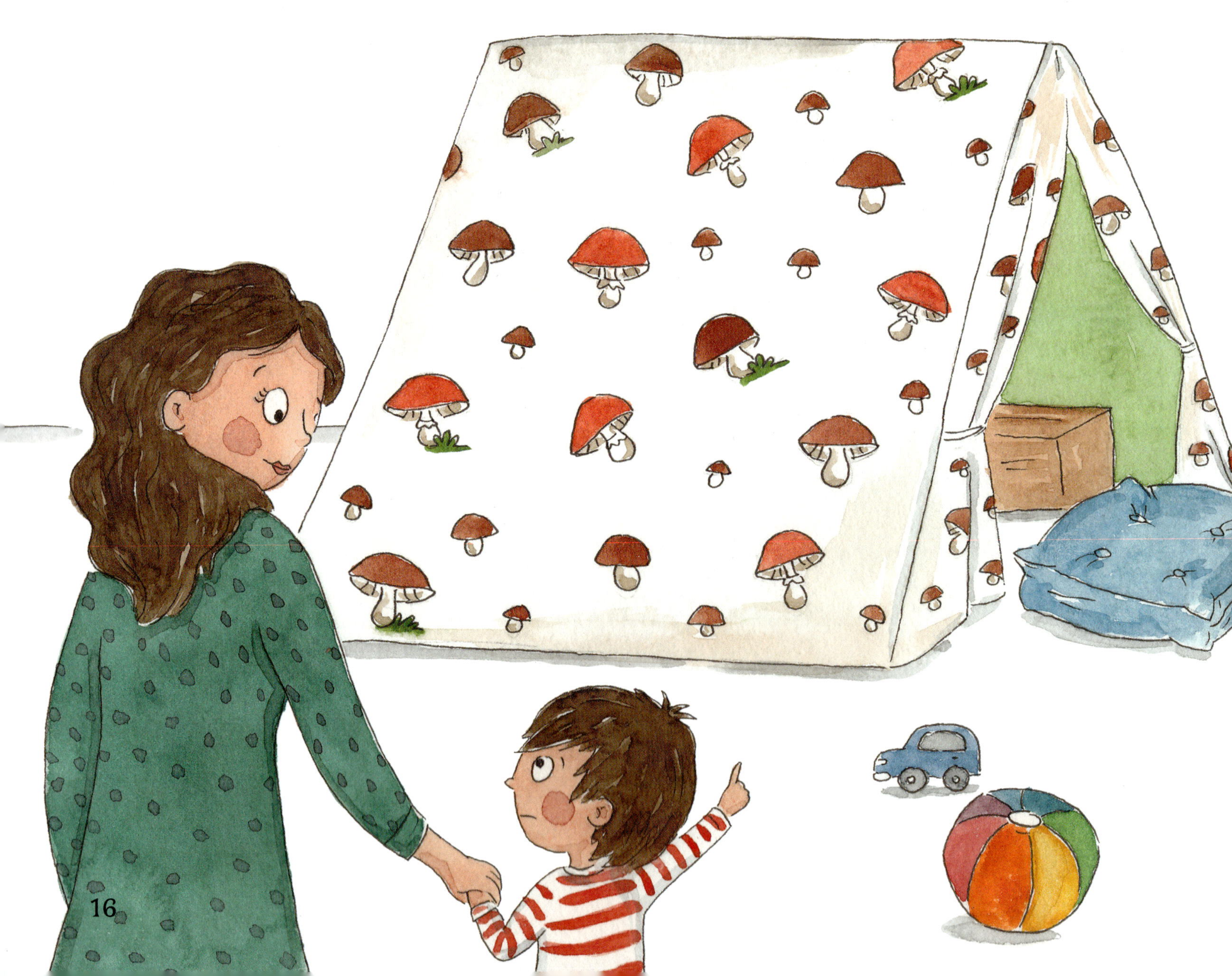

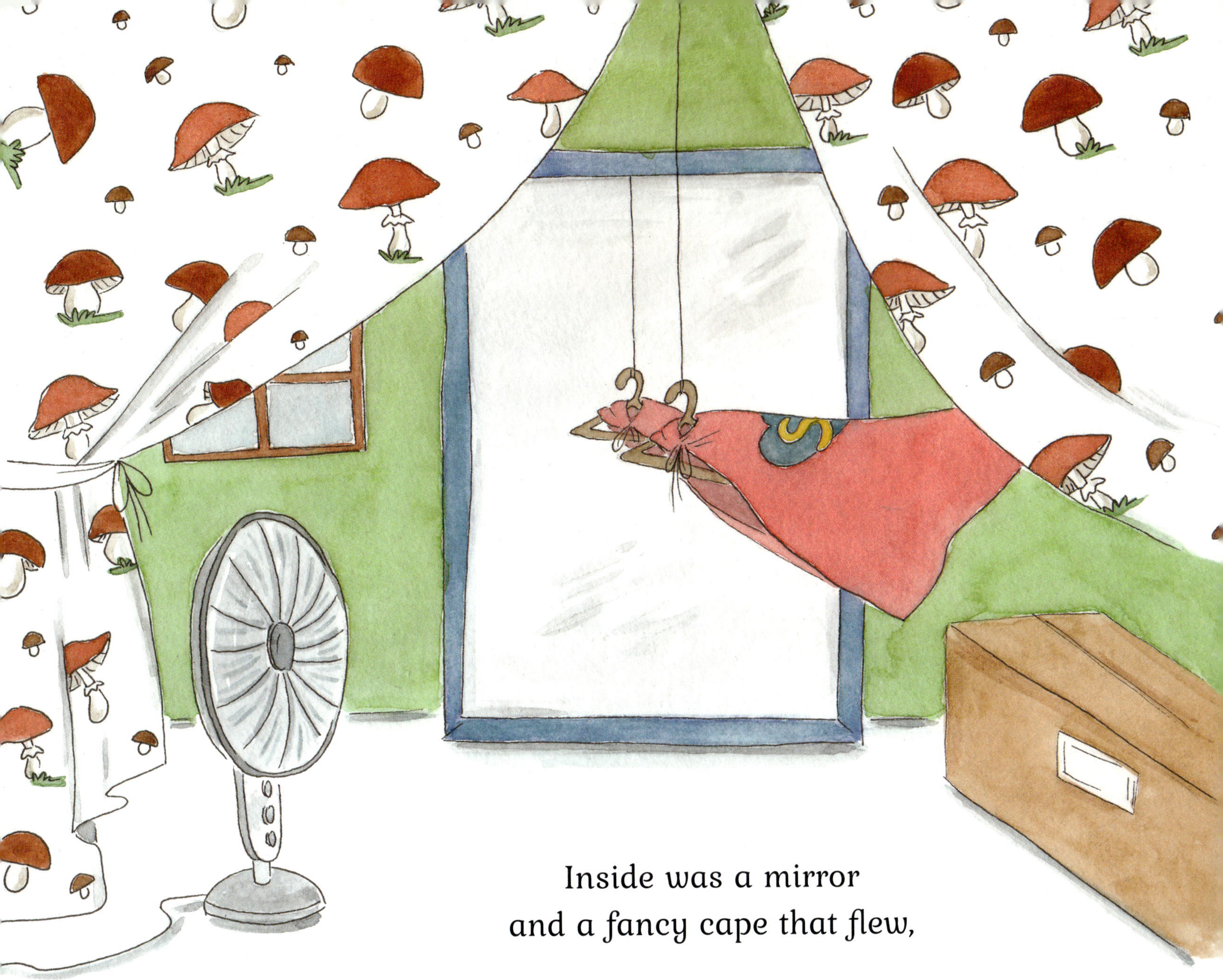

Inside was a mirror
and a fancy cape that flew,

‘For you always have to
protect your brother,’
said Mummy,
‘Your baby brother Andrew.’

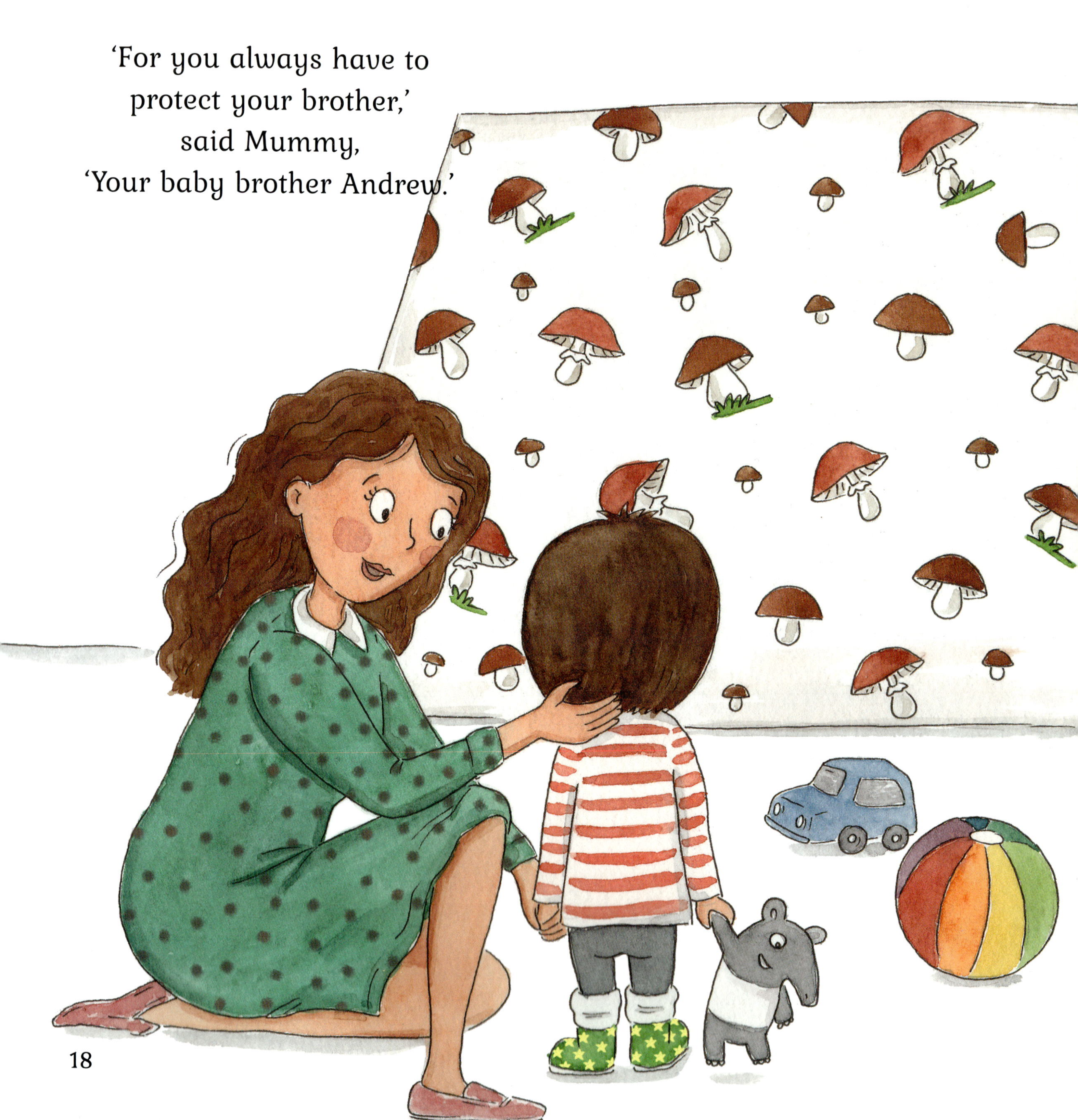

I was happy I had someone,
someone who was my own.
I couldn't wait to show my friends
what a cute little baby came,

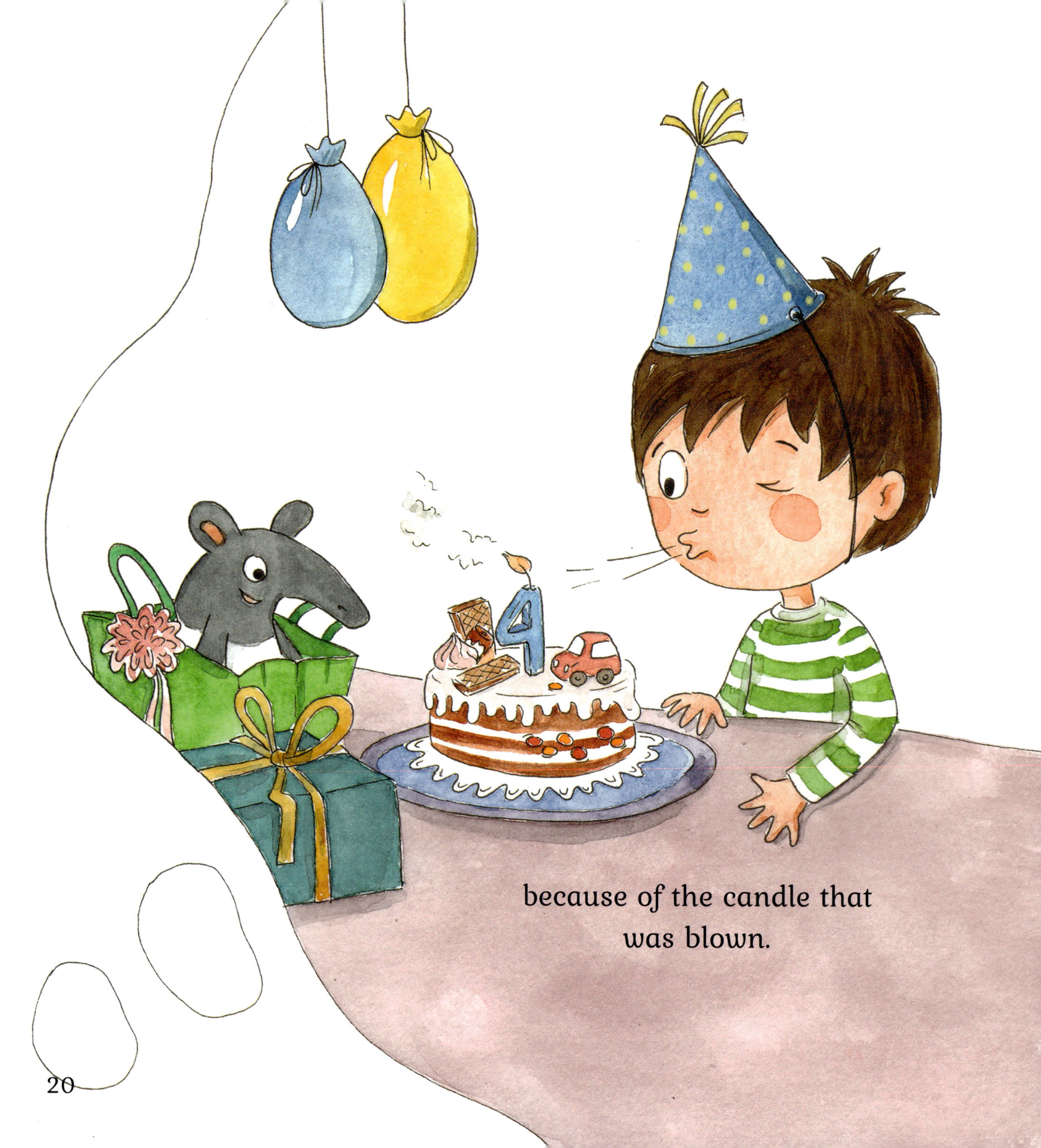

because of the candle that
was blown.

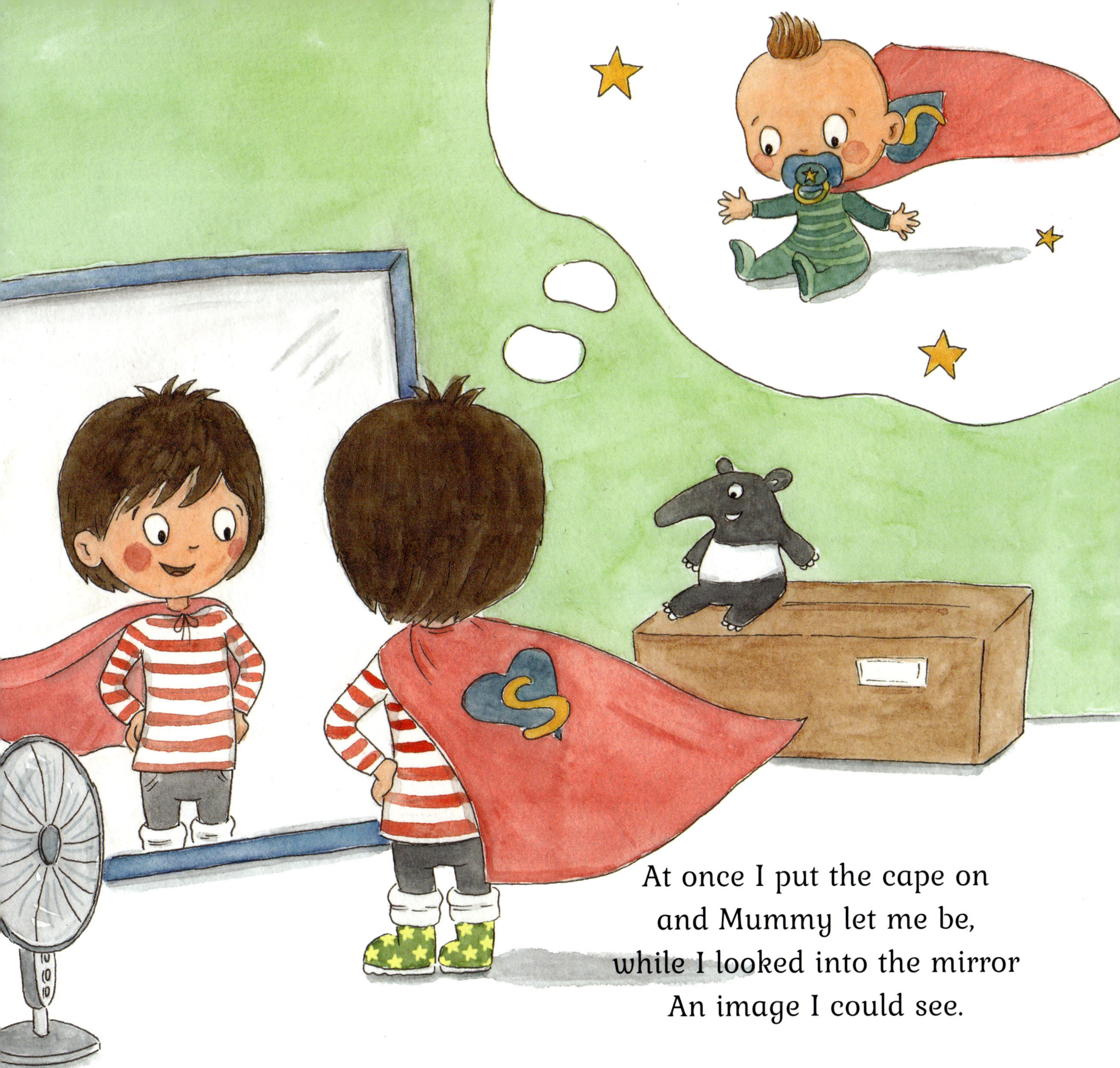

At once I put the cape on
and Mummy let me be,
while I looked into the mirror
An image I could see.

So I took the water colours
And painted the Muslin red

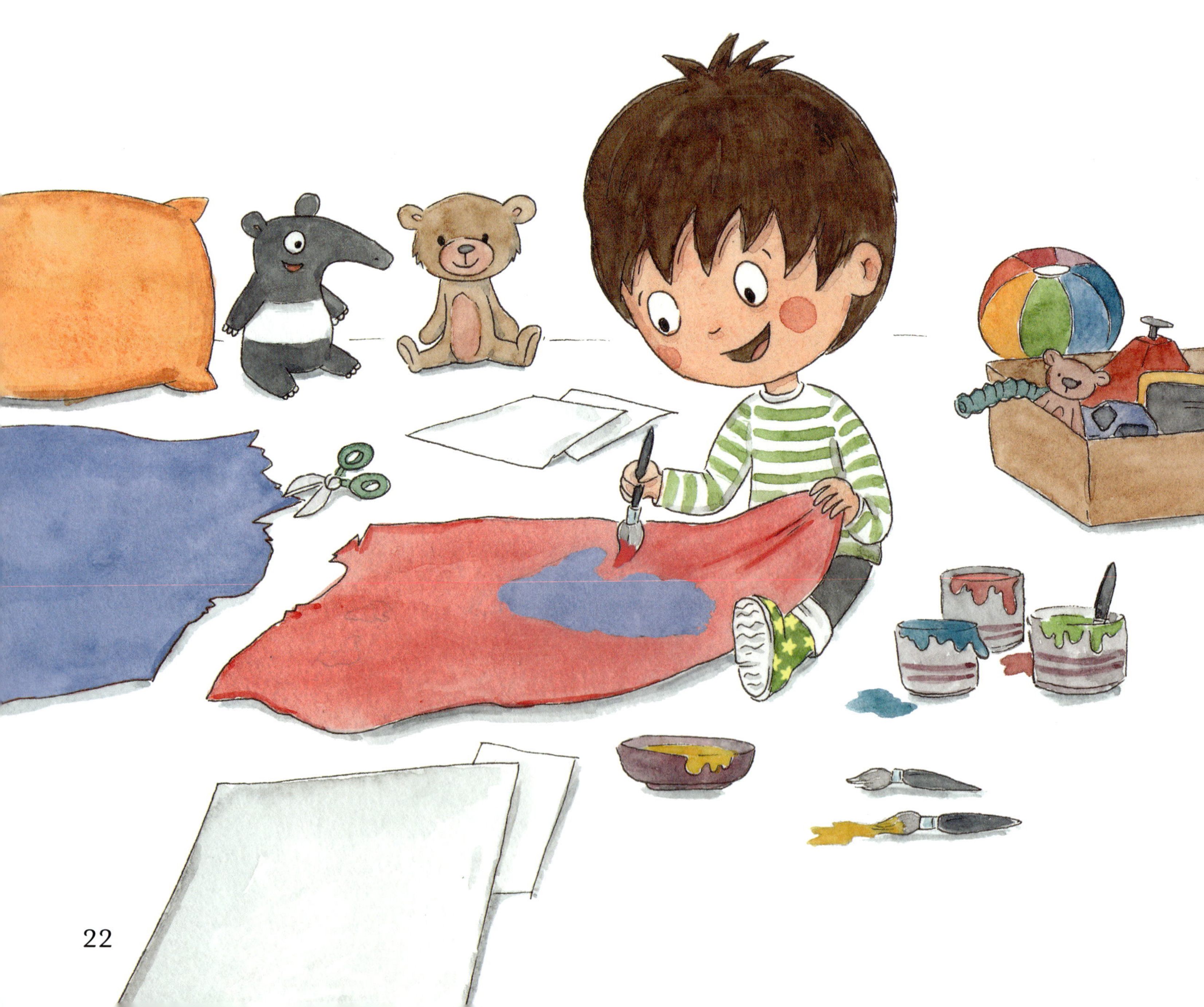

And marched up to
Andrew
To tie it round his
neck.

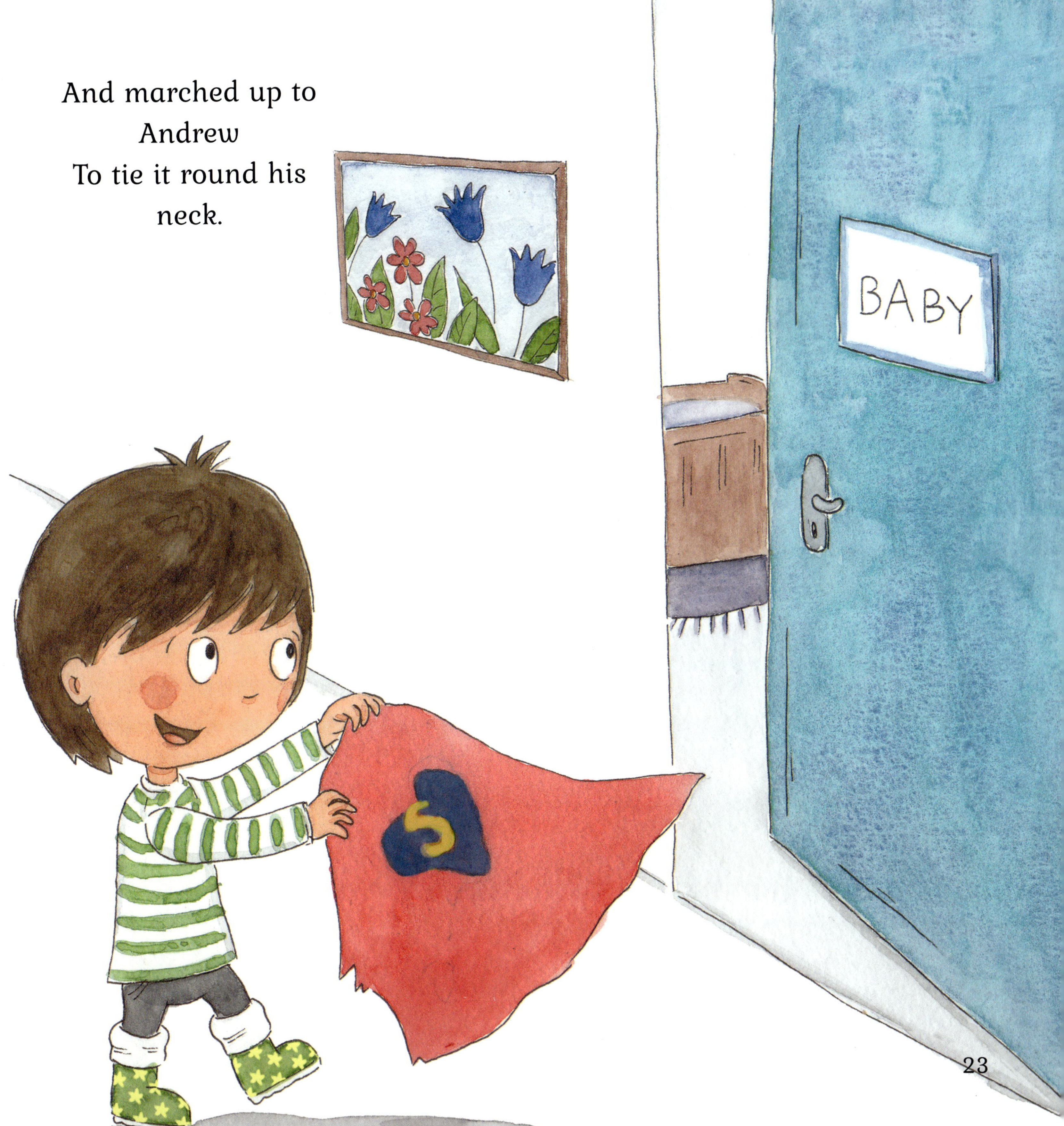

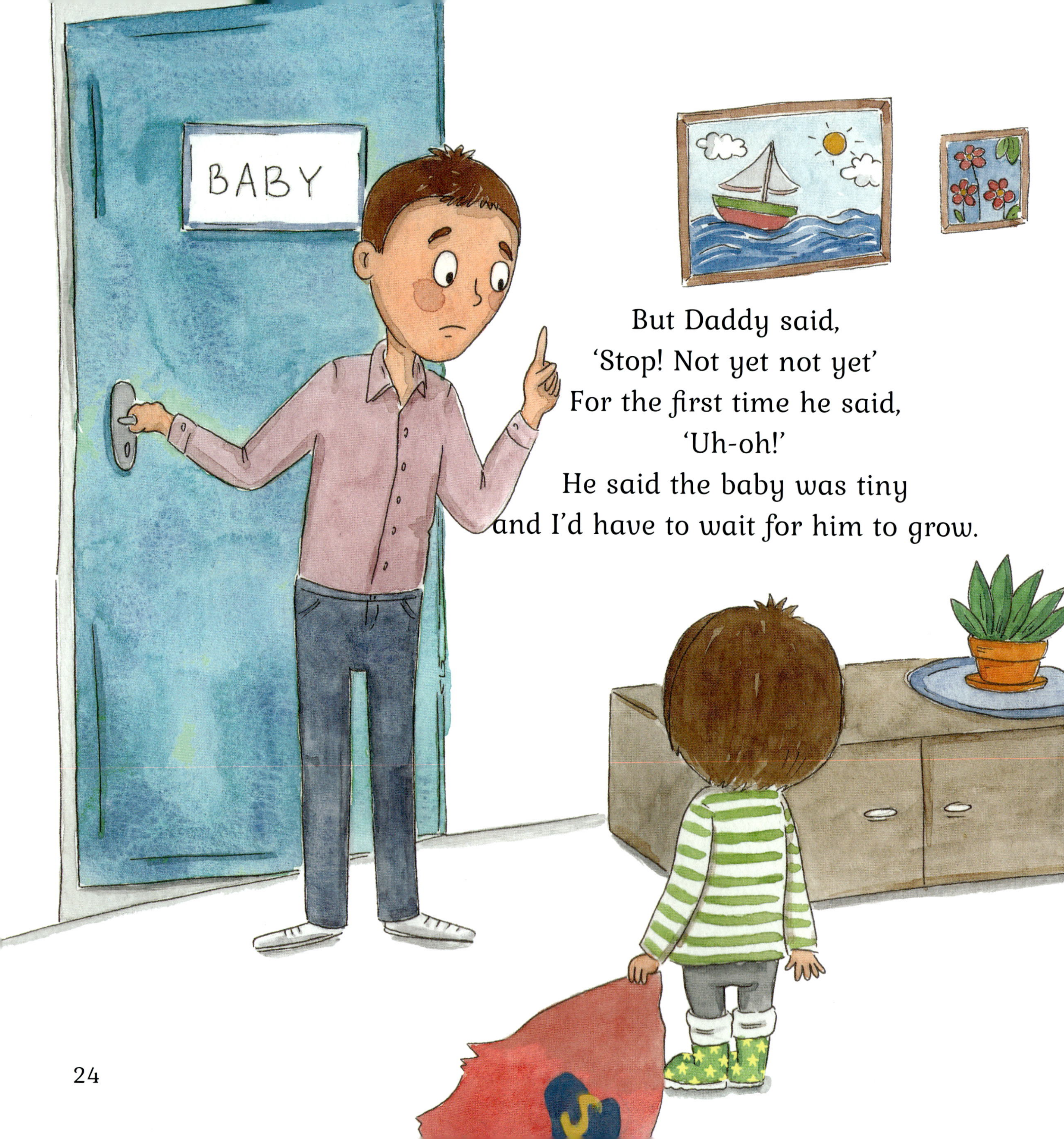

But Daddy said,
'Stop! Not yet not yet'
For the first time he said,
'Uh-oh!'
He said the baby was tiny
and I'd have to wait for him to grow.

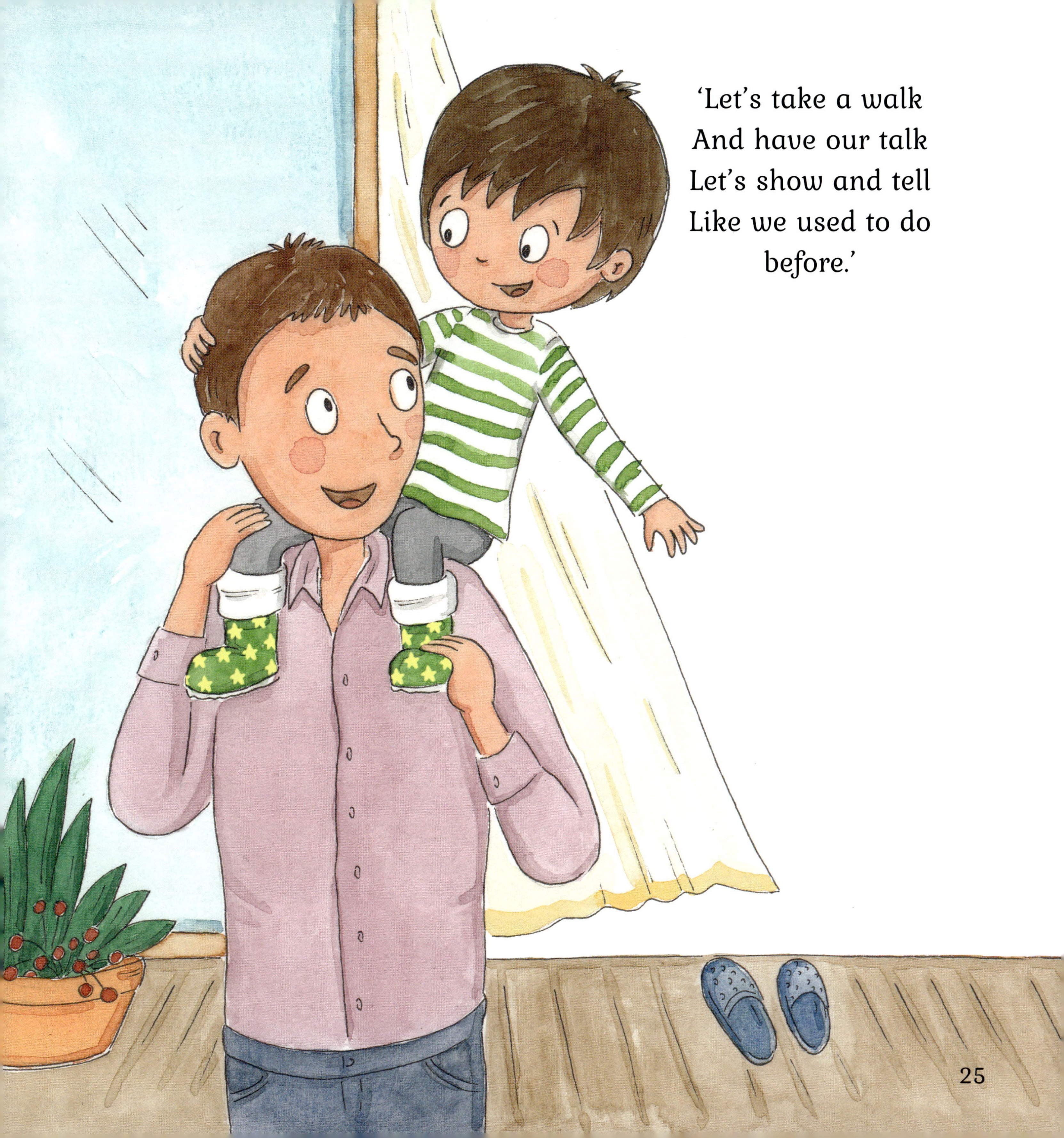

'Let's take a walk
And have our talk
Let's show and tell
Like we used to do
before.'

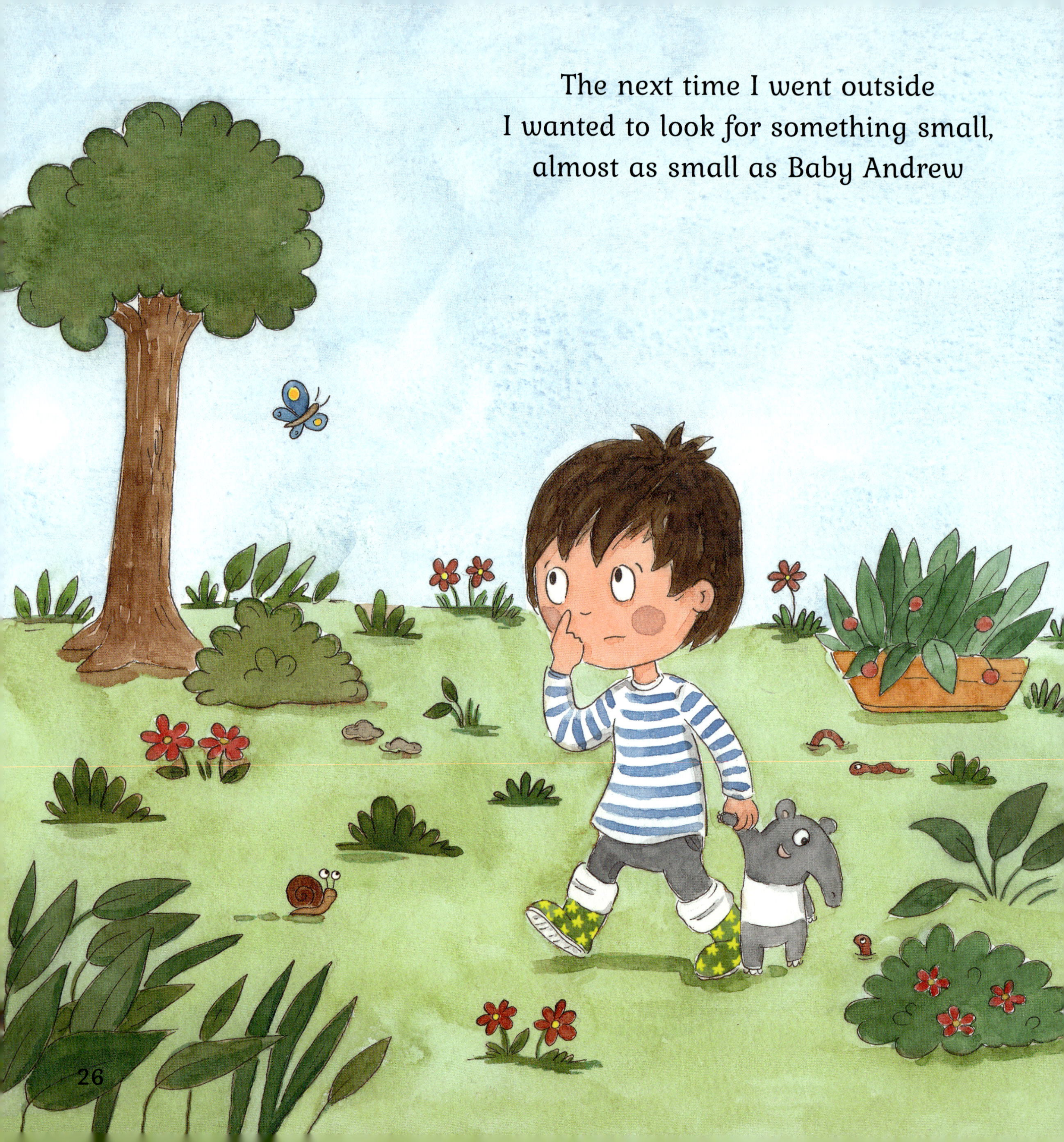

The next time I went outside
I wanted to look for something small,
almost as small as Baby Andrew

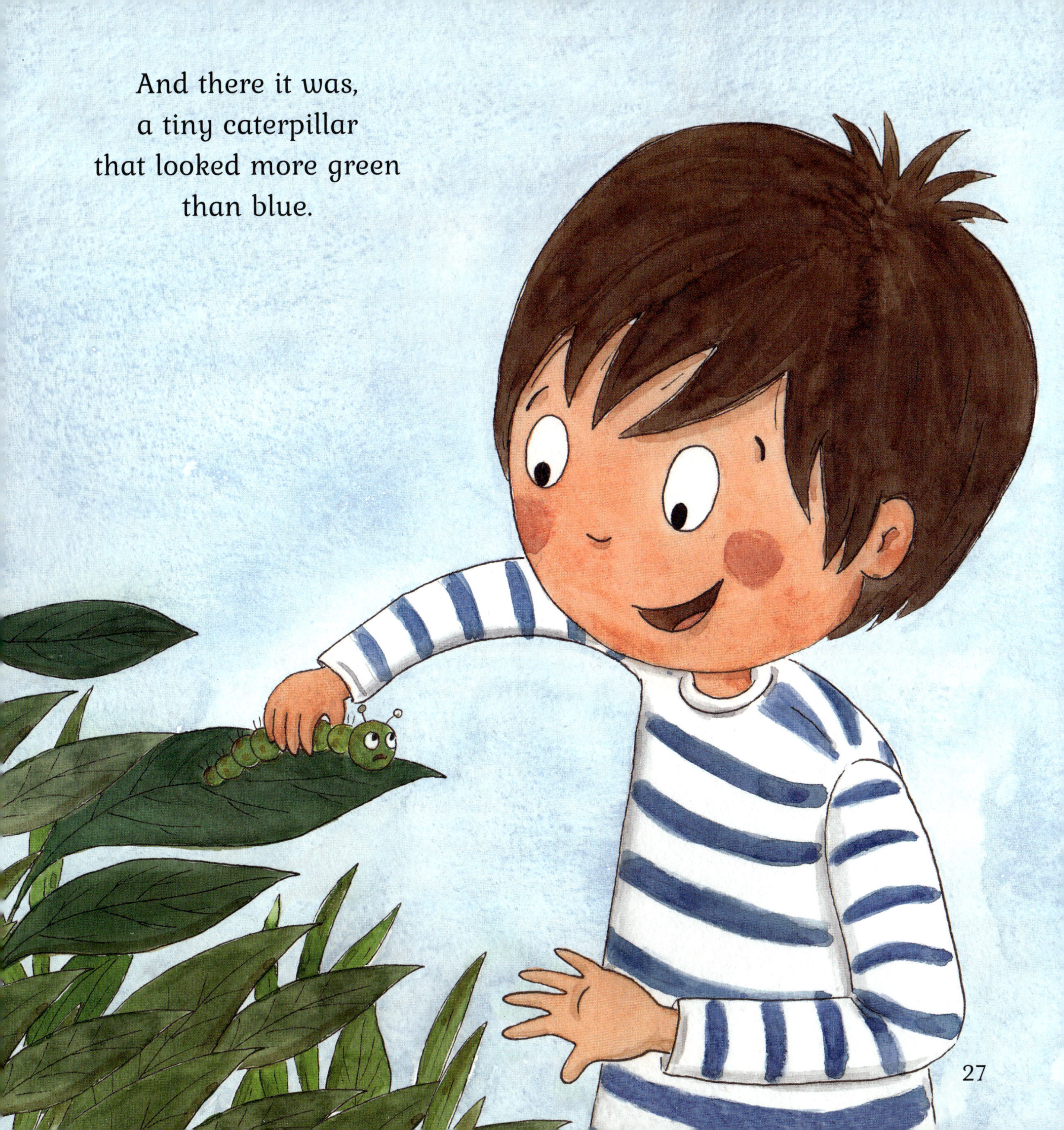

And there it was,
a tiny caterpillar
that looked more green
than blue.

But Grandpa said
'Stop! Not yet not yet'
For the first time he said
'Uh-oh!'

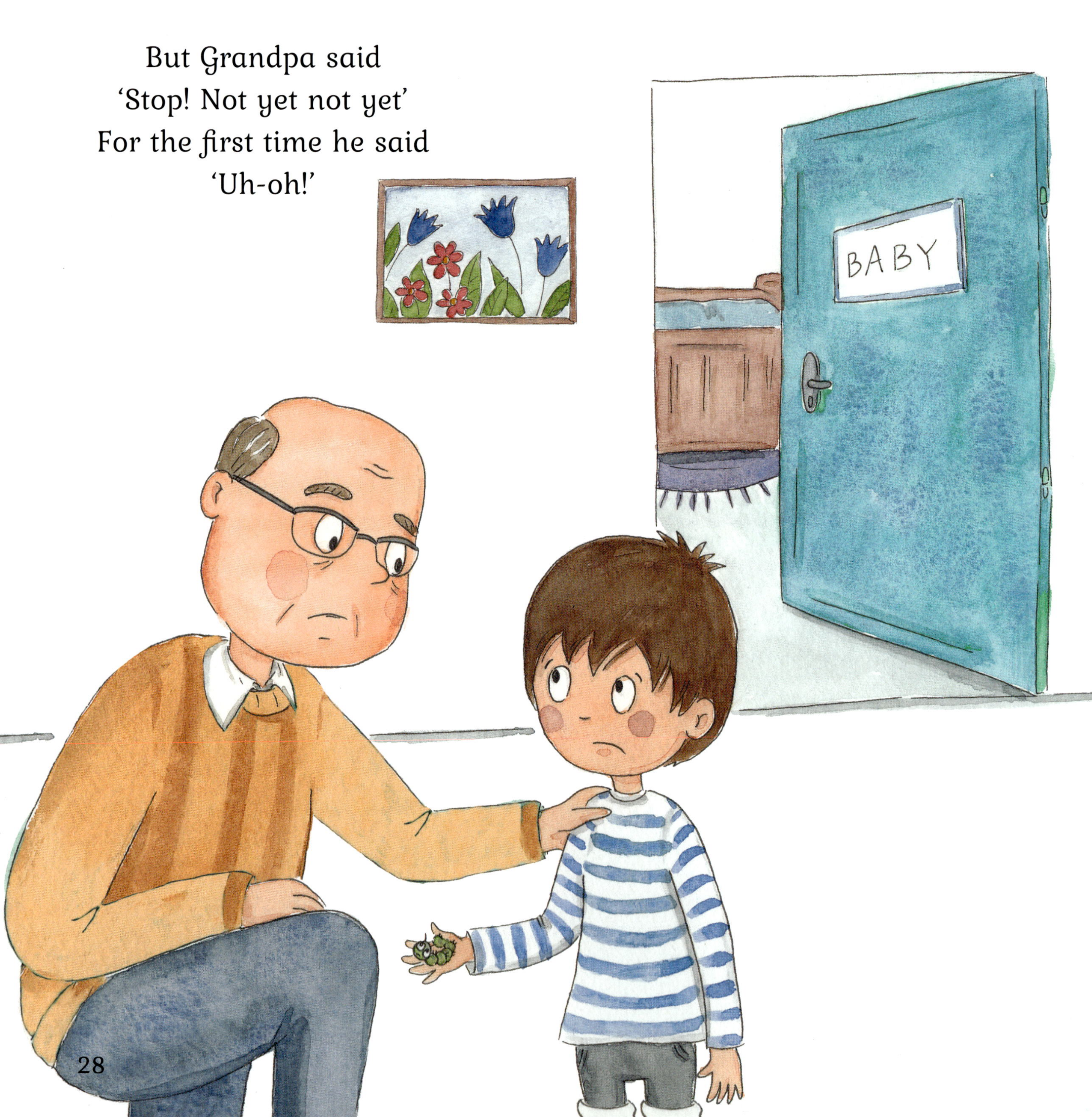

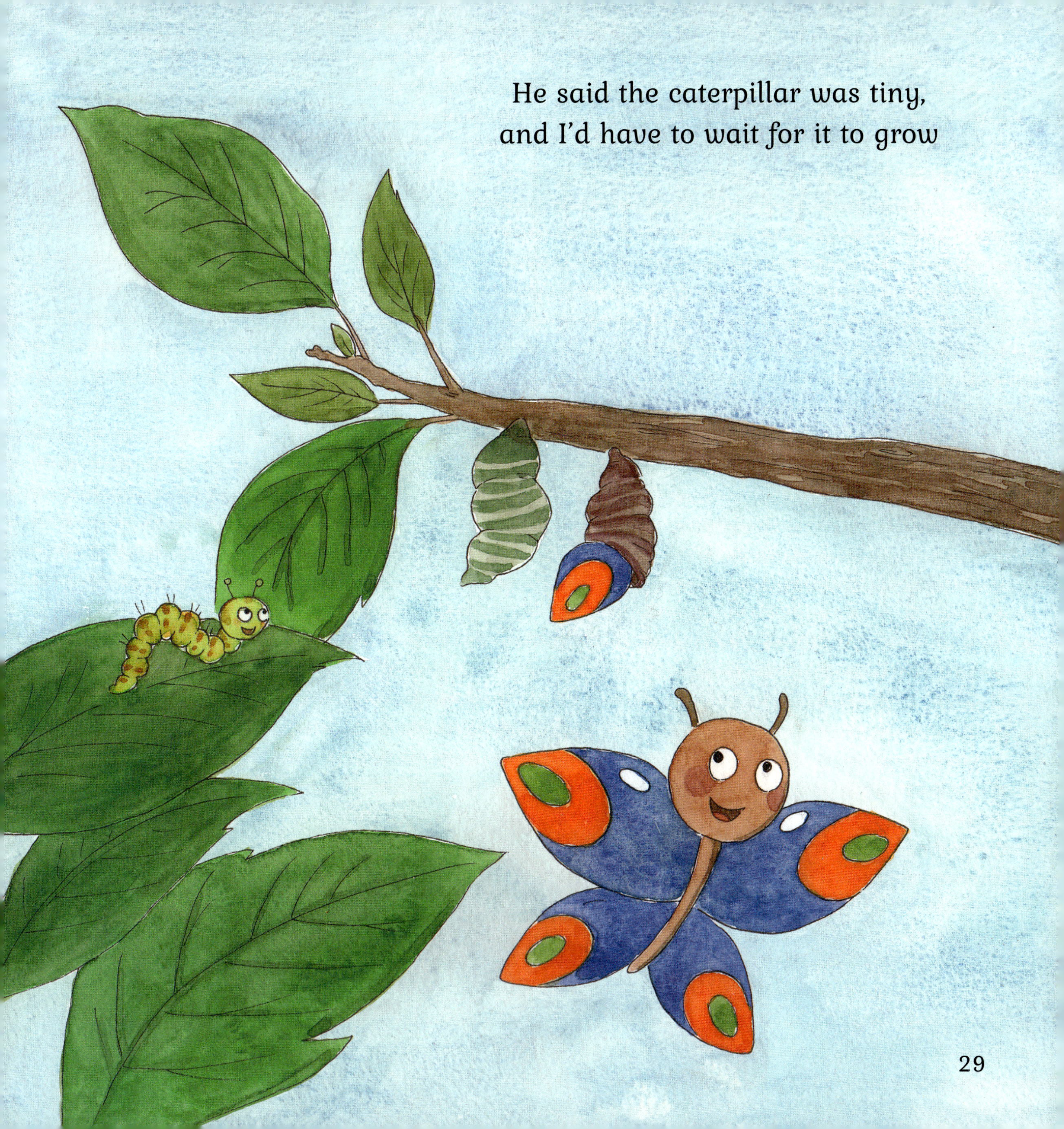

He said the caterpillar was tiny,
and I'd have to wait for it to grow

'You come with me
and play with me
the game we always play,
here take my glasses and
put them back on
in your topsy-turvy way.'

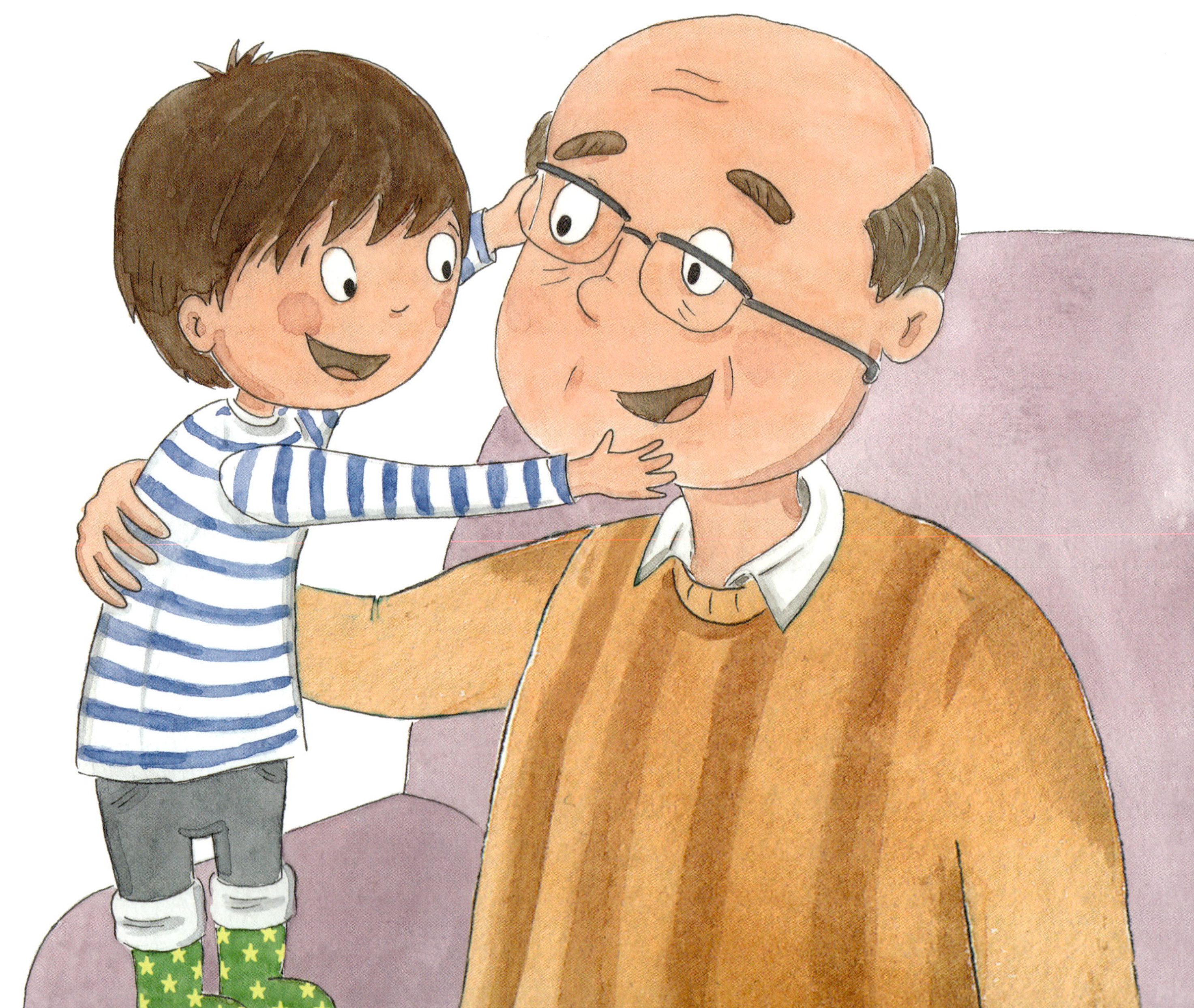

Few weeks later
I walked around
to find something delish,
I stopped in front of a bowl of
glass
that had some water and fish.

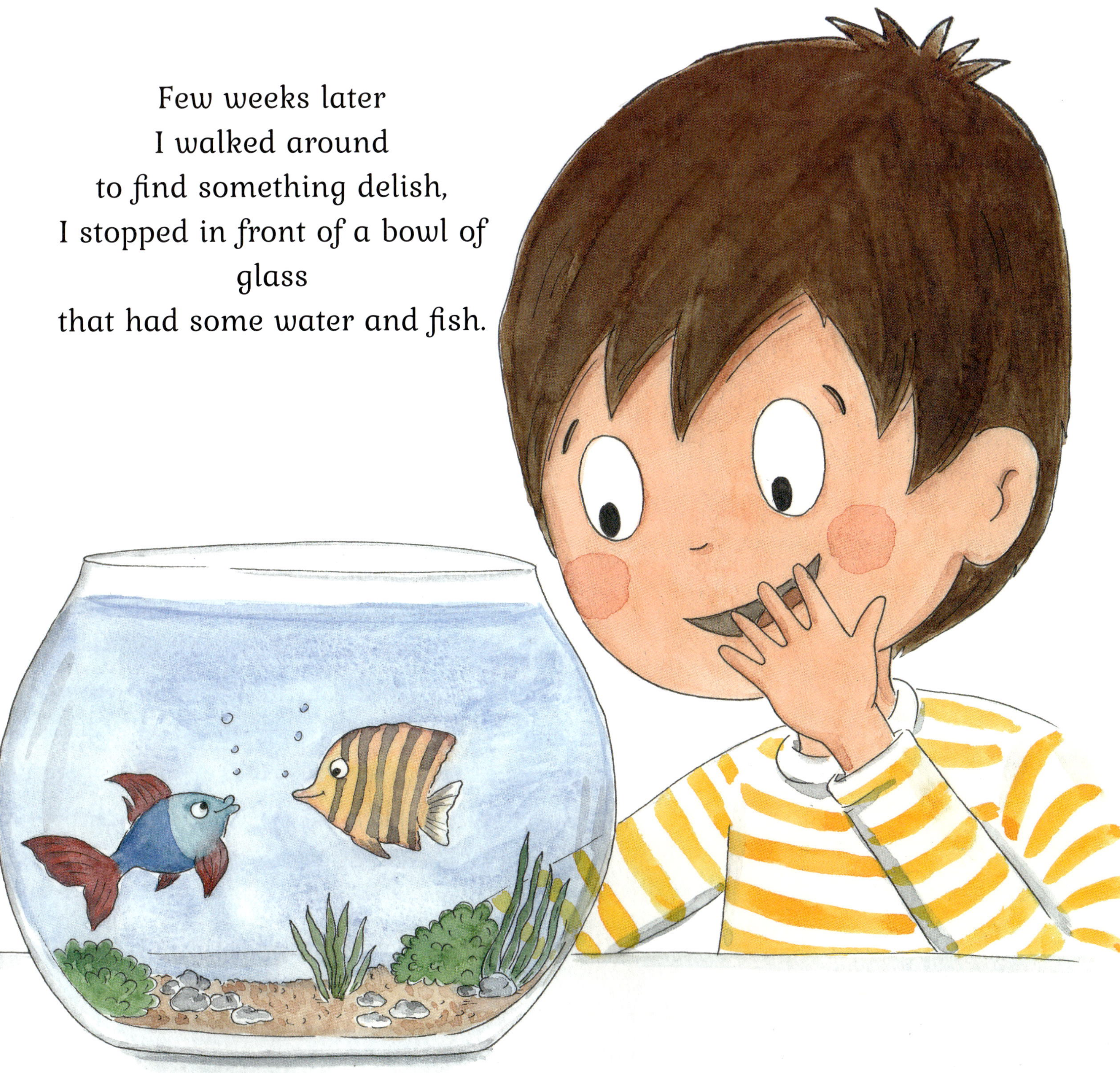

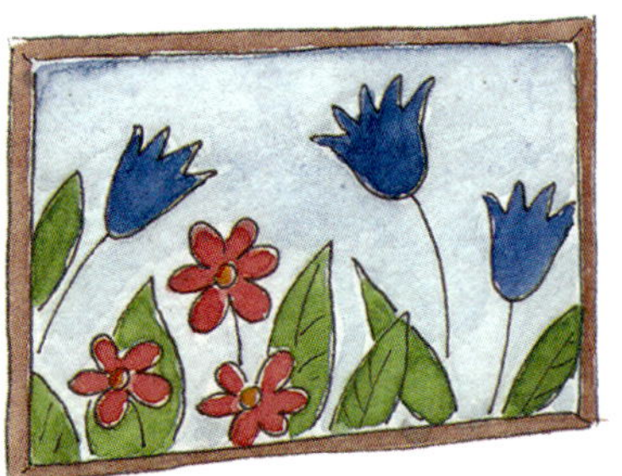

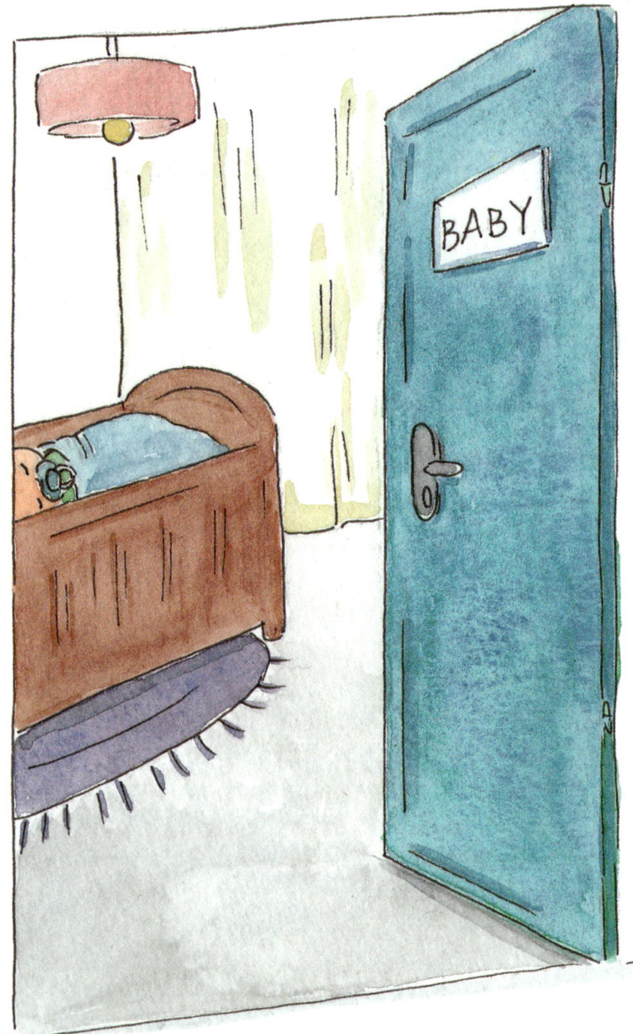

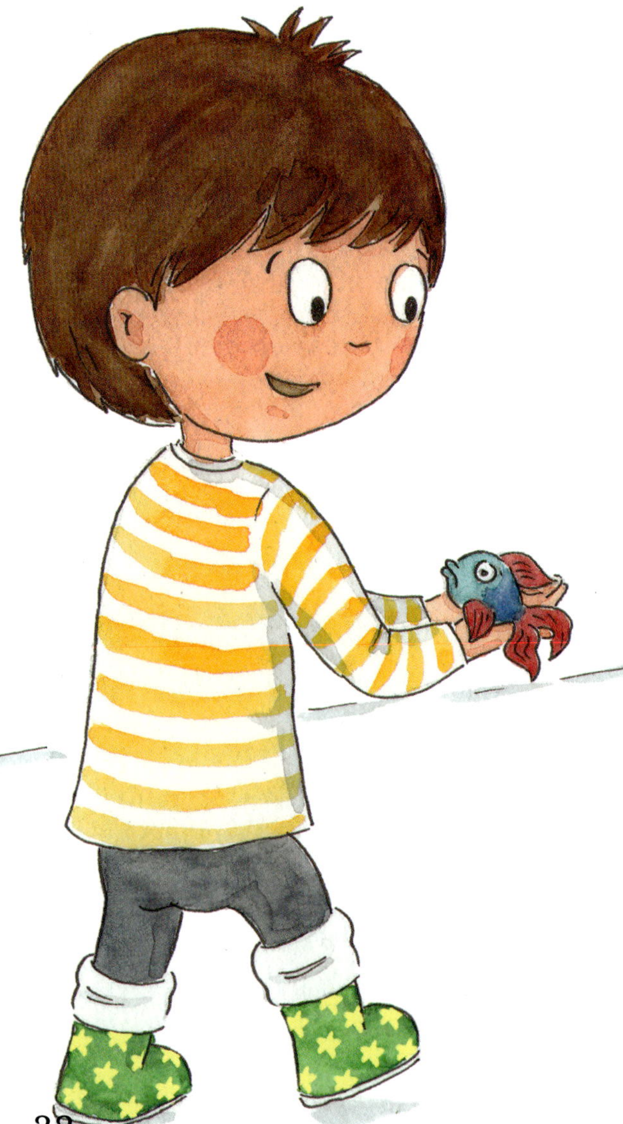

And just like that
I reached for it,
It wiggled in my palm like slime.
I walked up to the room again
I was sure this time
my idea would shine.

But Grandma said
'Stop! Not yet not yet'
For the first time she said,
'UH-oh!'

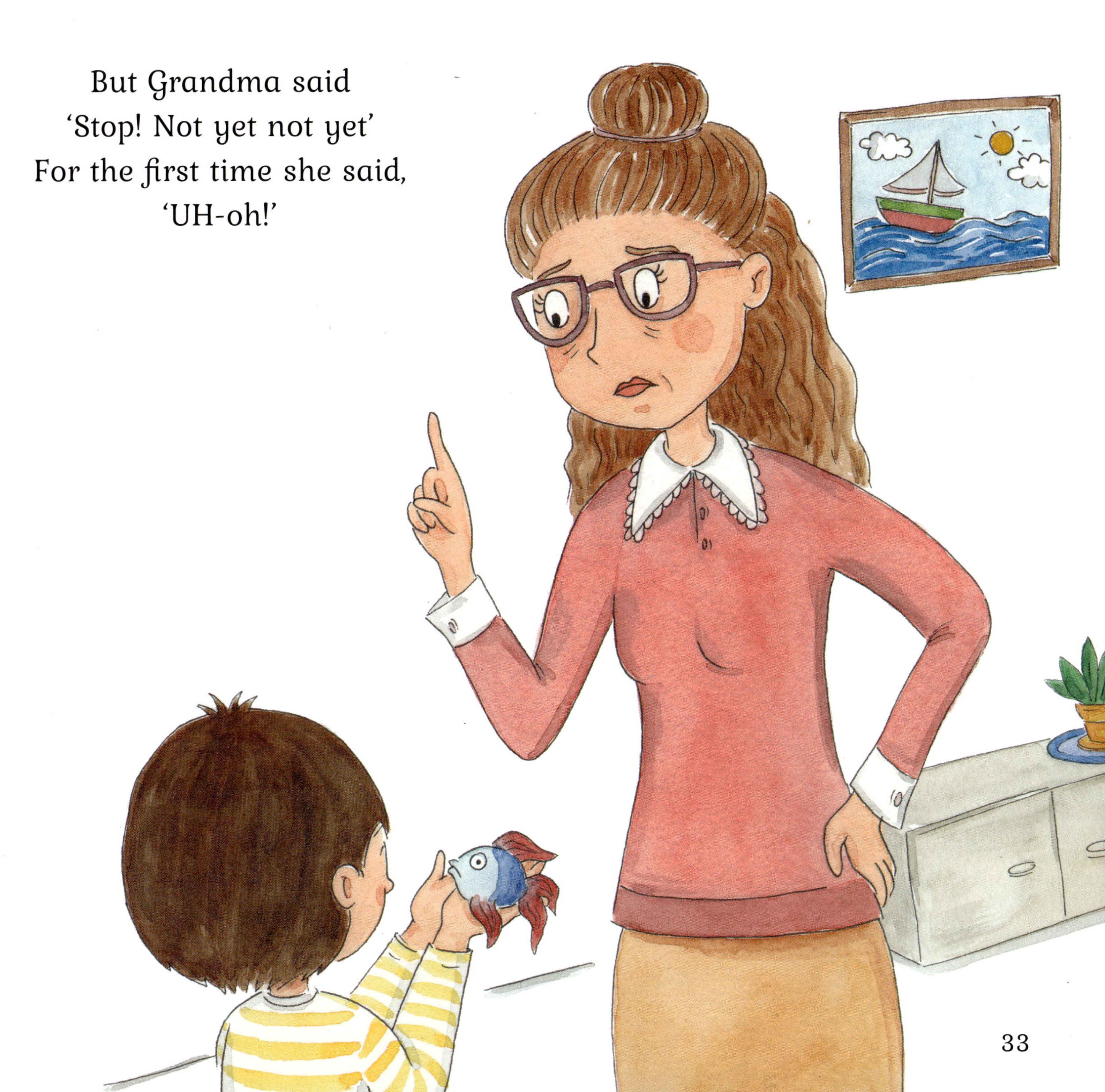

She said the baby was tiny,
and I'd have to wait for him to grow.

'You come with me
Let's bake a cake
I'll let you lick the spoon.

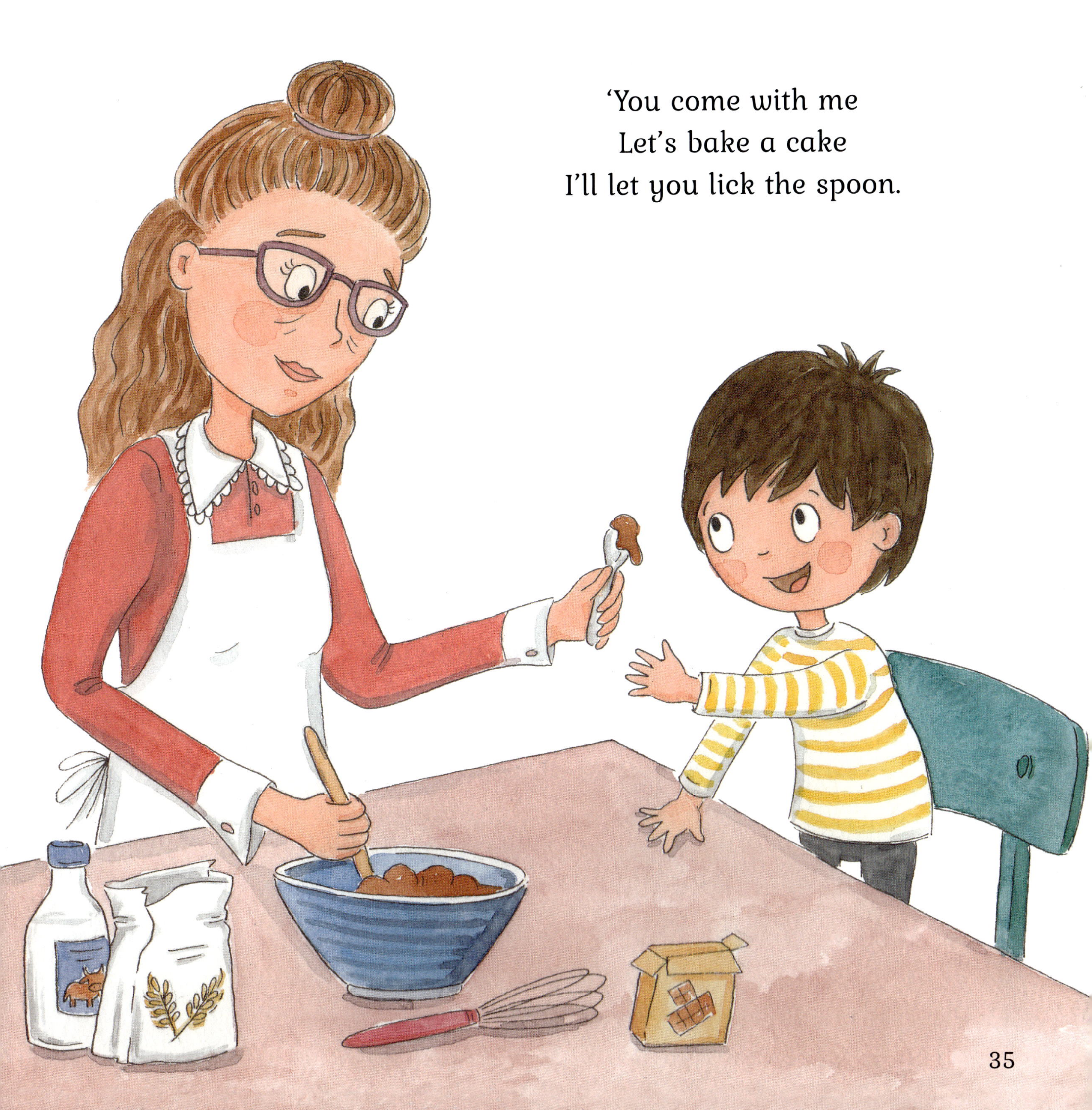

As days go by,
you'll have your turn
to play with Andrew,
very soon.'

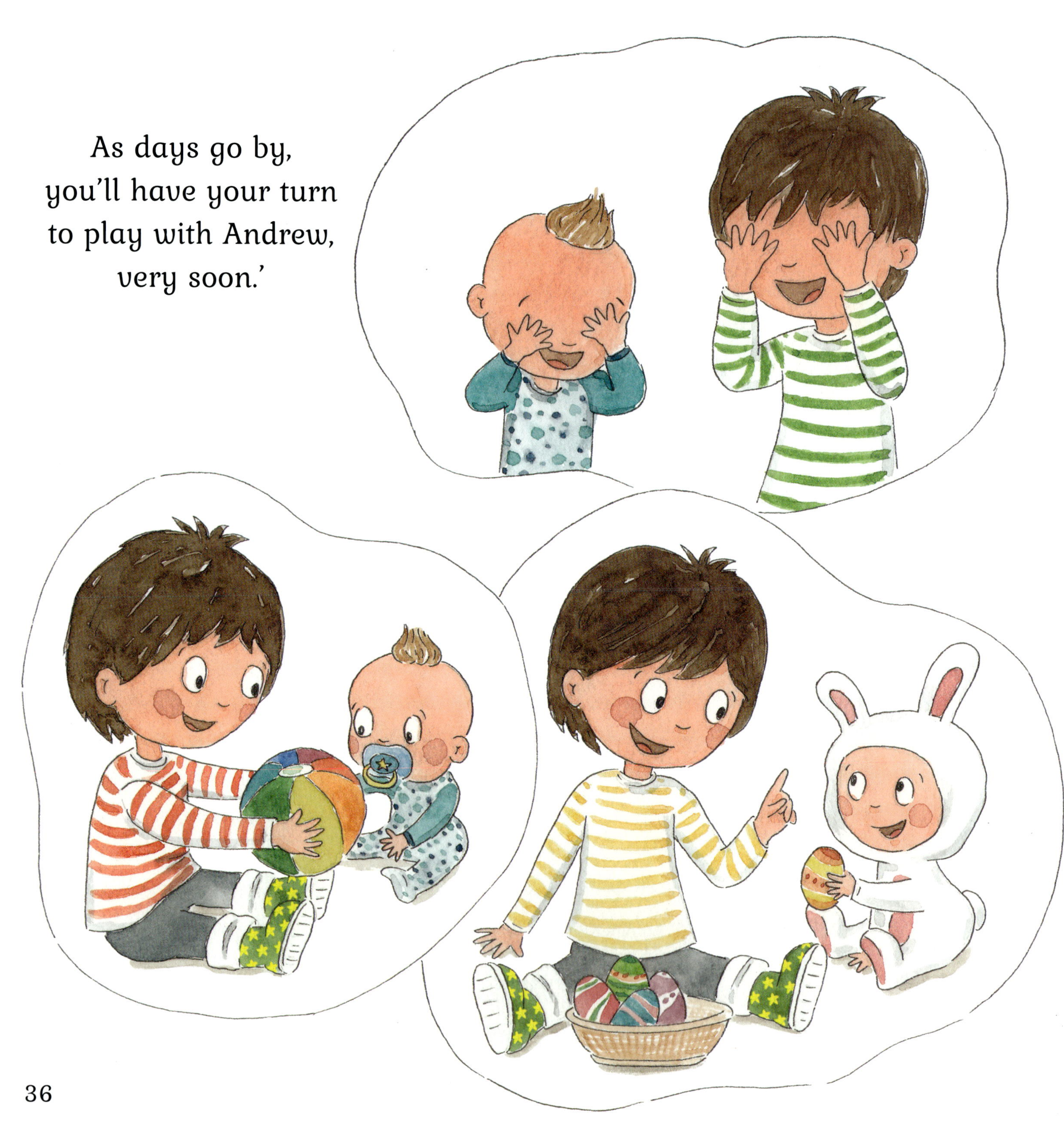

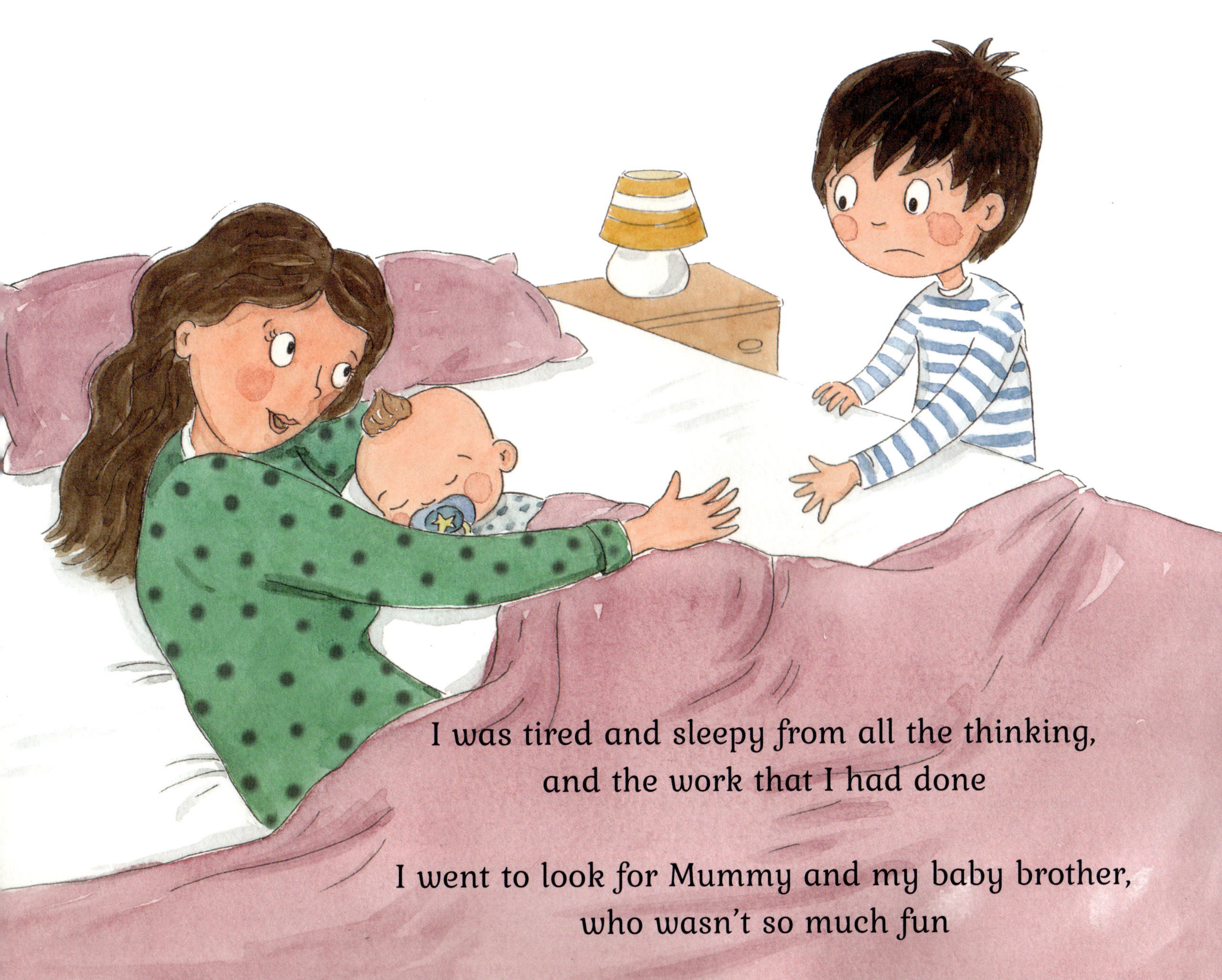

I was tired and sleepy from all the thinking,
and the work that I had done

I went to look for Mummy and my baby brother,
who wasn't so much fun

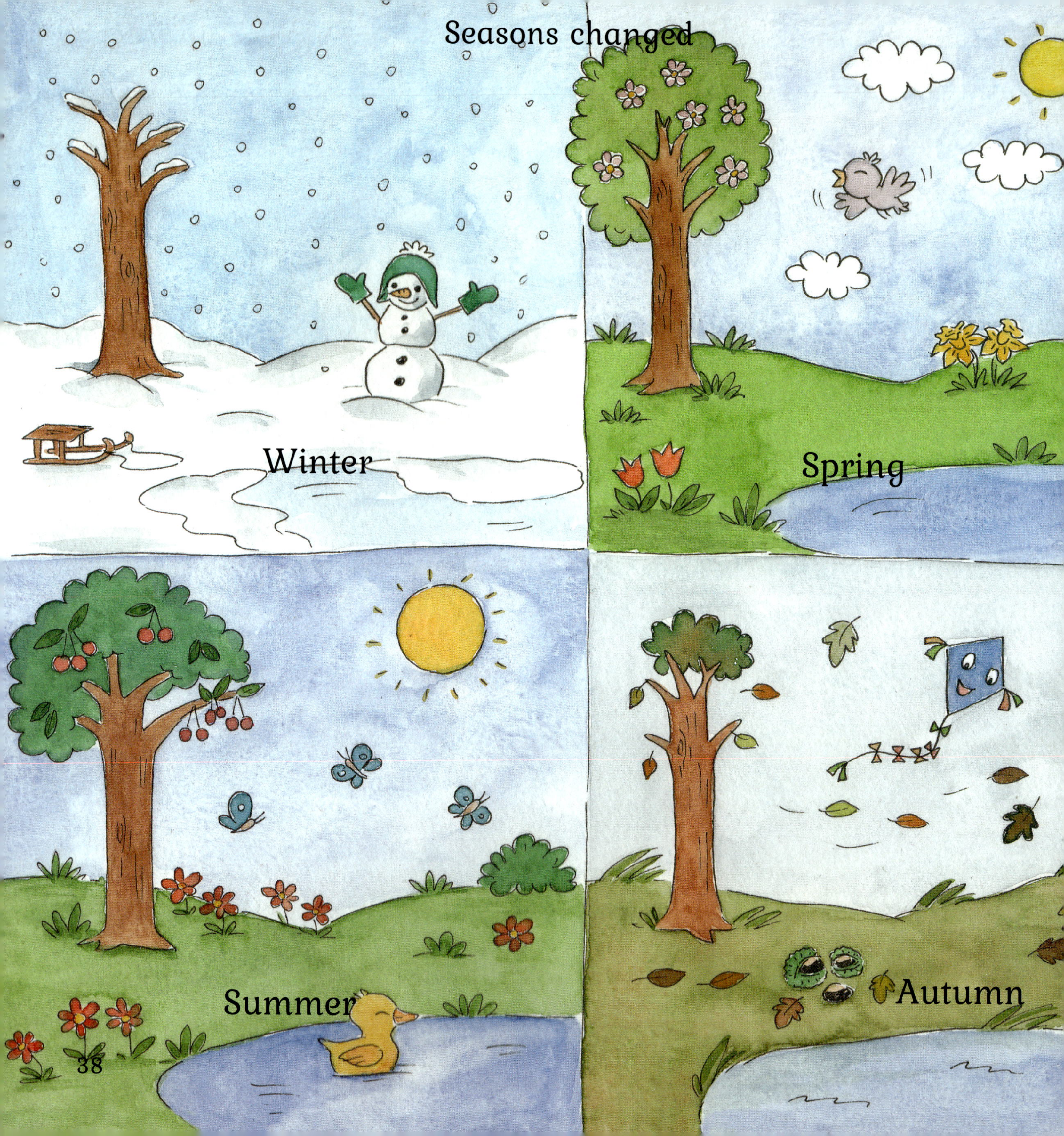
Seasons changed
Winter
Spring
Summer
Autumn

And so did I

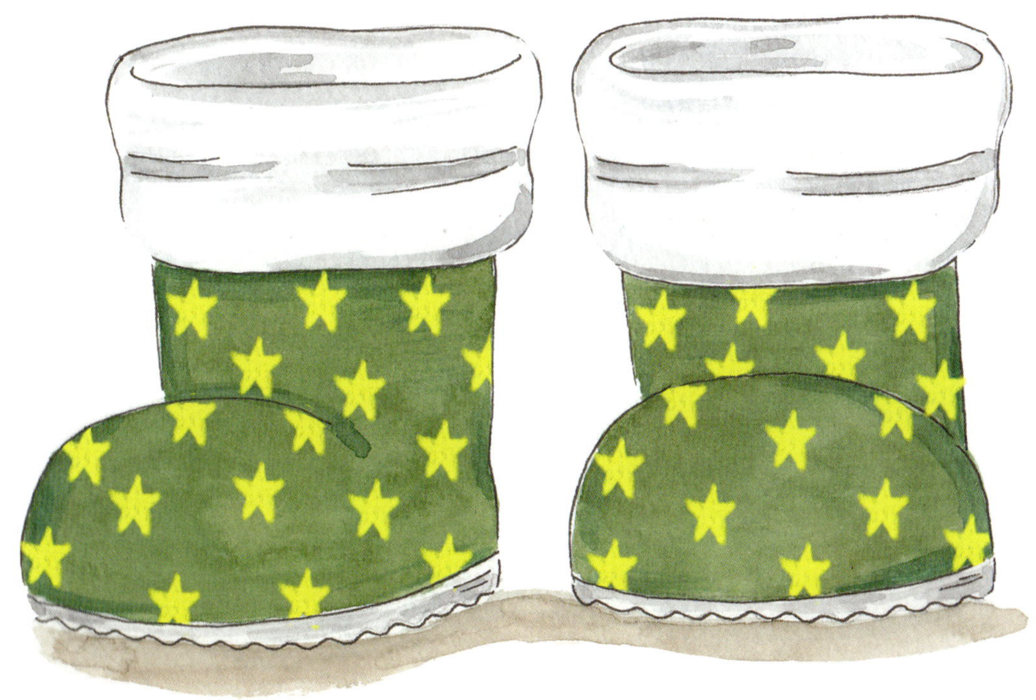

My feet were now big for
my shoes

Sometimes we would
sleep together
Sometimes, Grandma and
Grandpa with Andrew

Then one morning
I felt a kick
and woke up with a grumpy face,
but Mummy had a big smile.
Andrew had climbed up on me
and crawled to the other side.

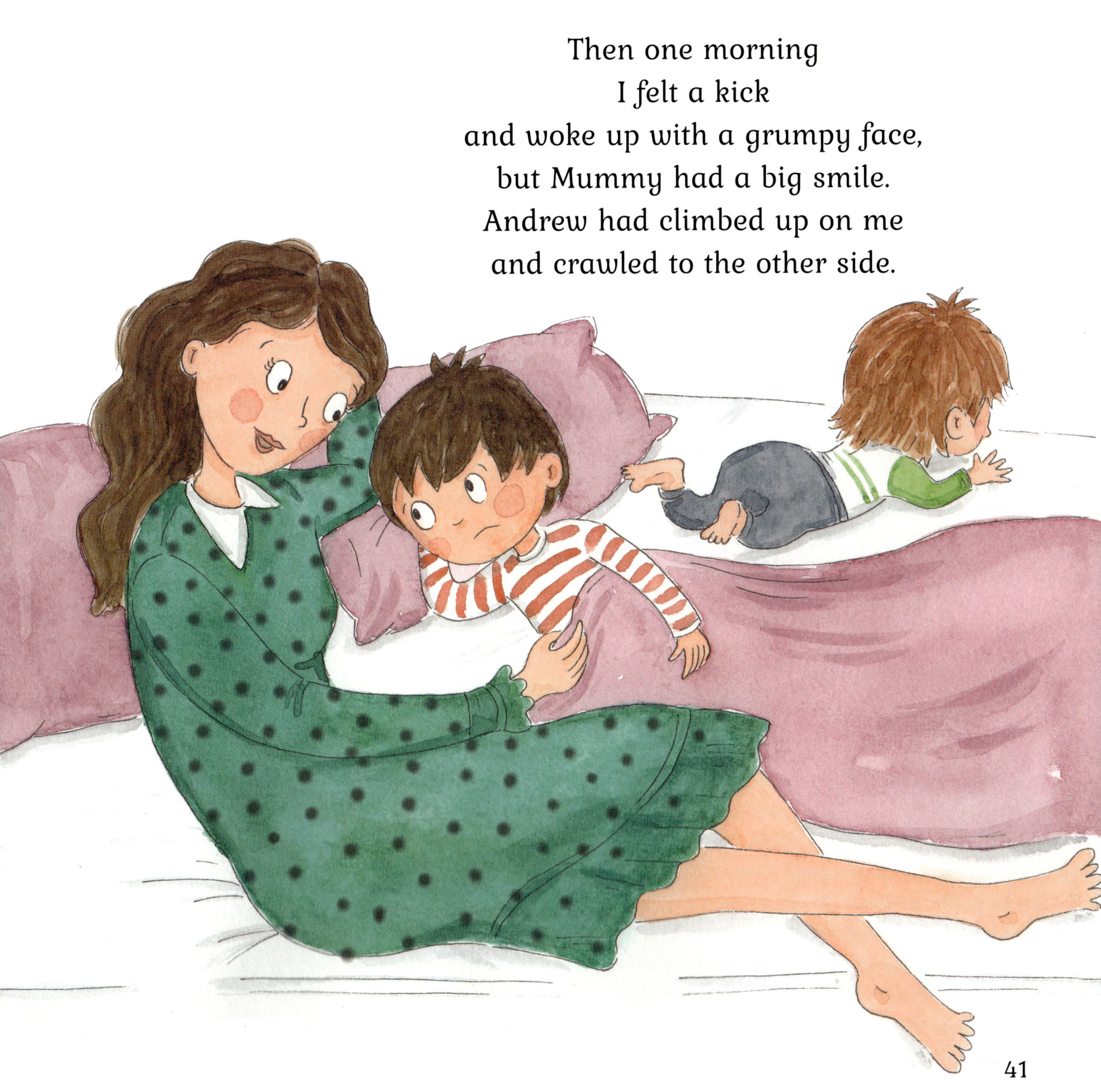

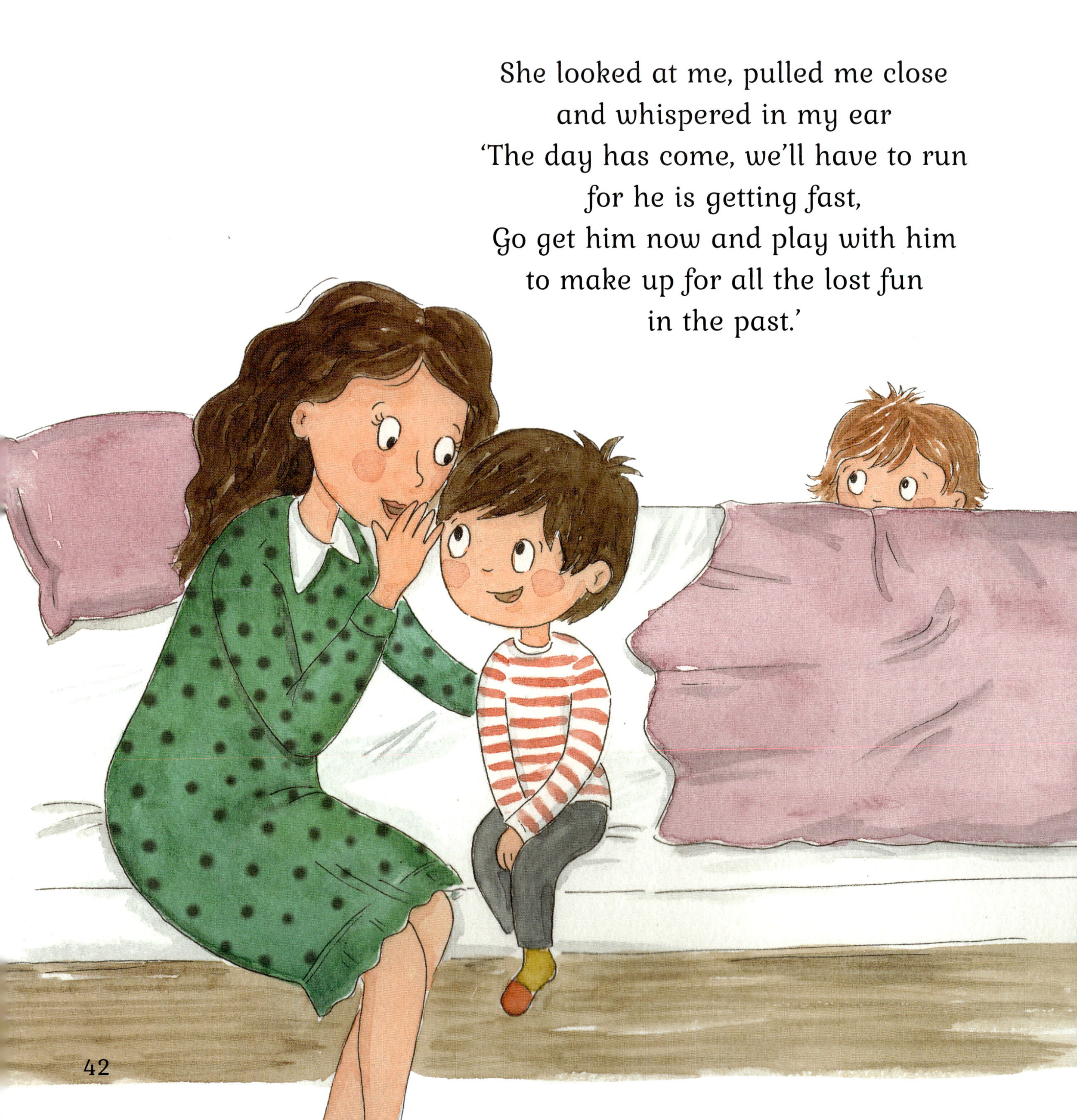

She looked at me, pulled me close
and whispered in my ear
'The day has come, we'll have to run
for he is getting fast,
Go get him now and play with him
to make up for all the lost fun
in the past.'

He crawled towards the curtain
and hid under the bed,
in the hope that
I would bend,

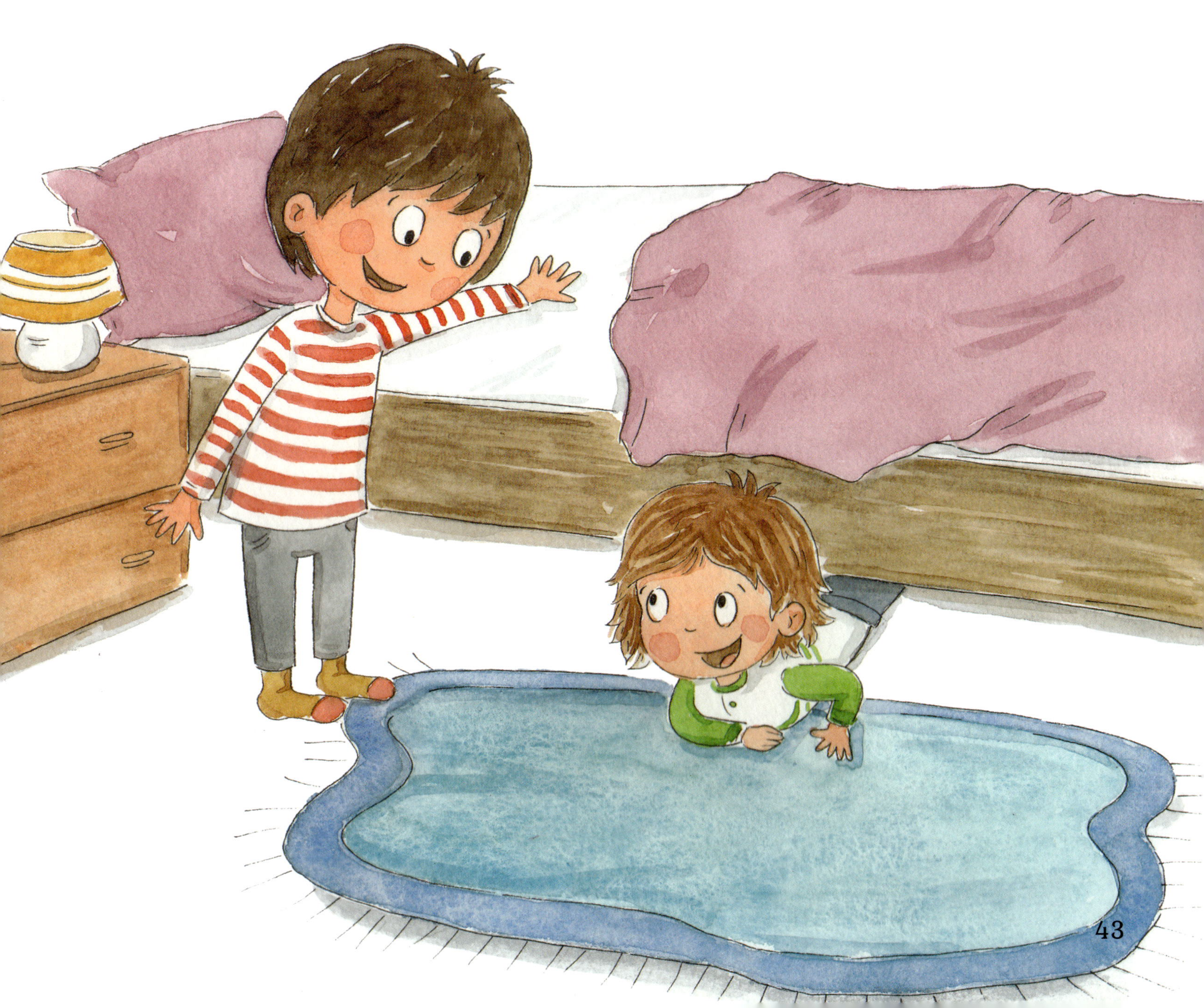

and that's the very day
My baby brother,
Became *my best friend!*

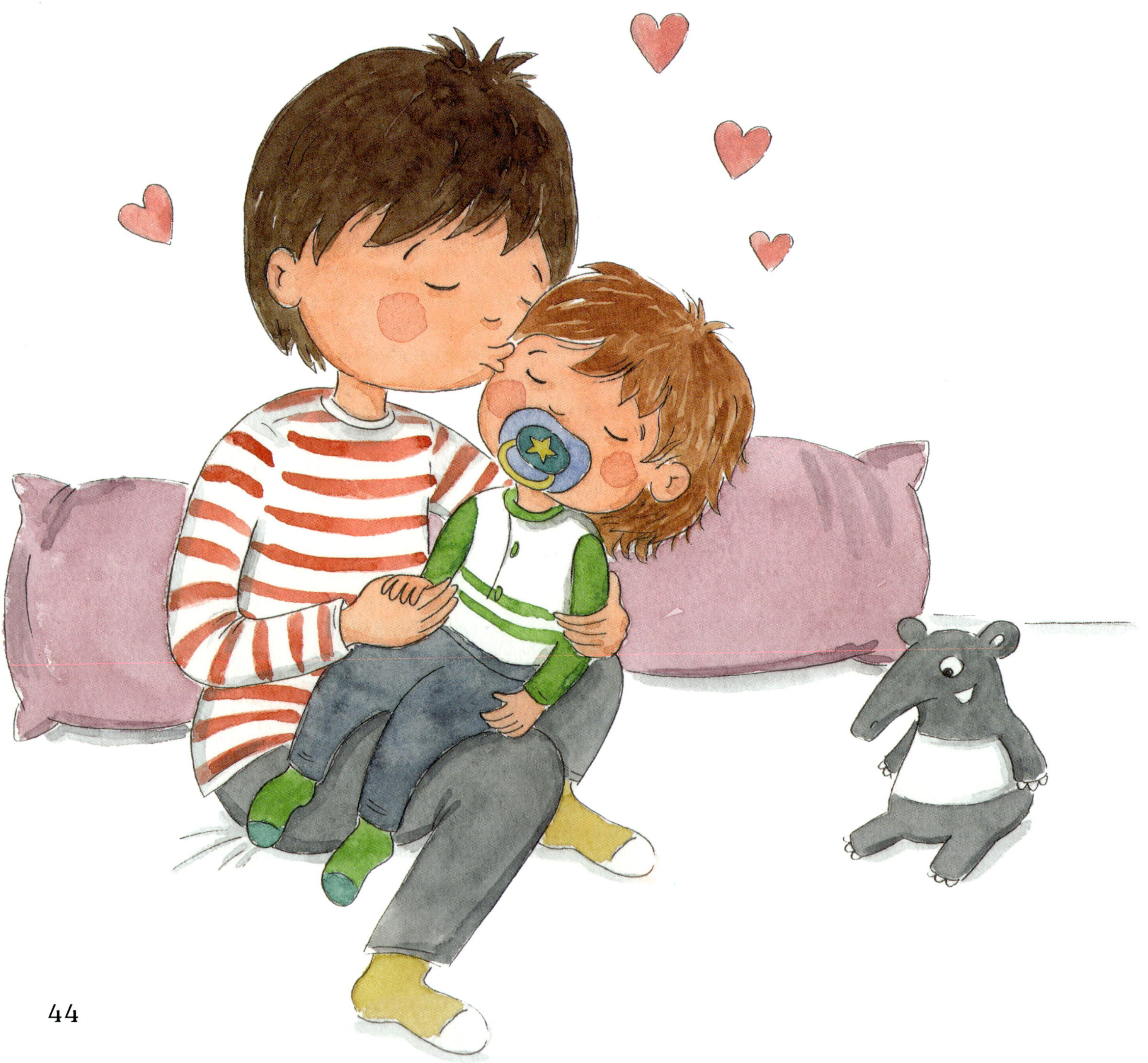

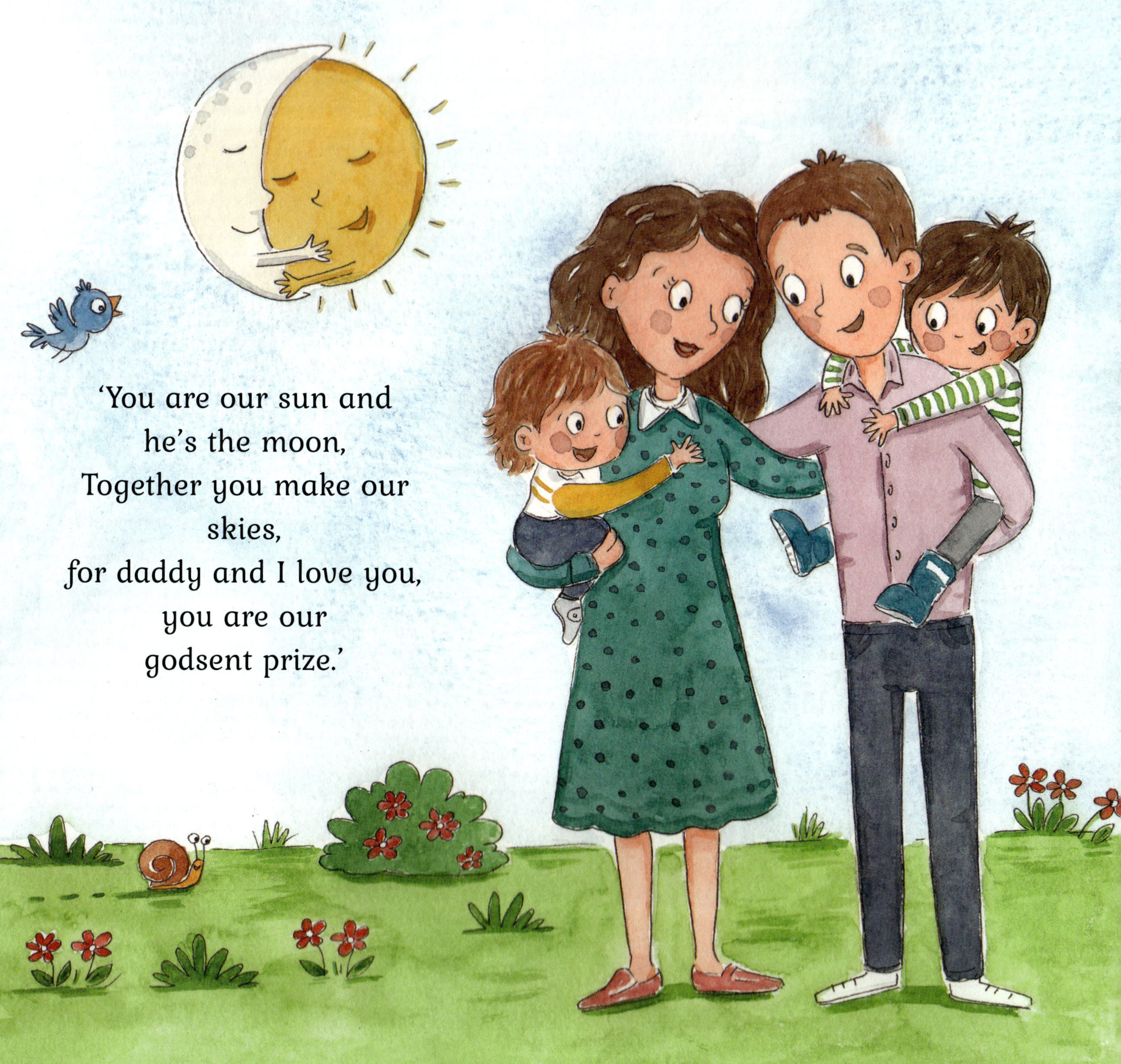

‘You are our sun and
he’s the moon,
Together you make our
skies,
for daddy and I love you,
you are our
godsent prize.’

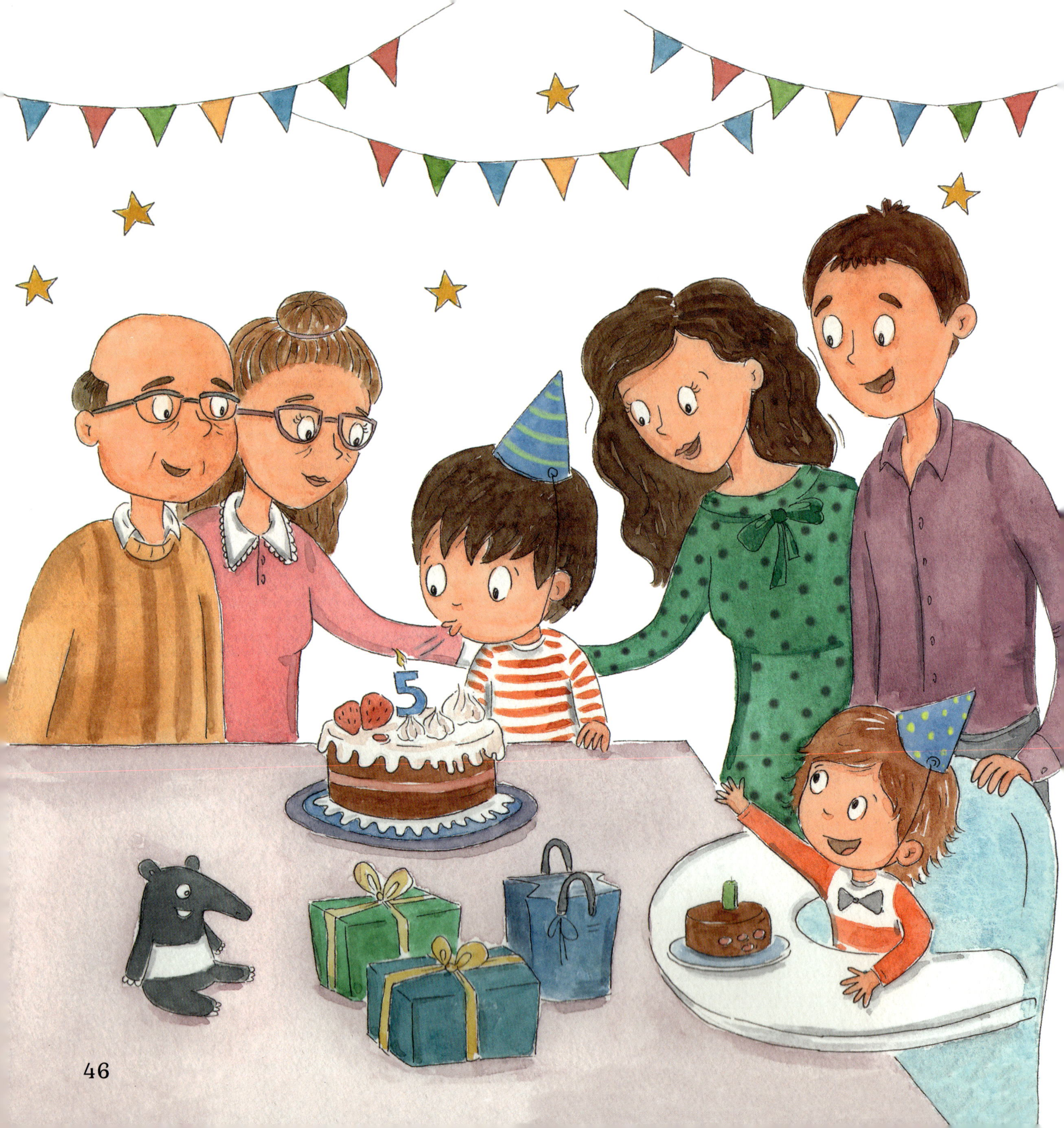
5

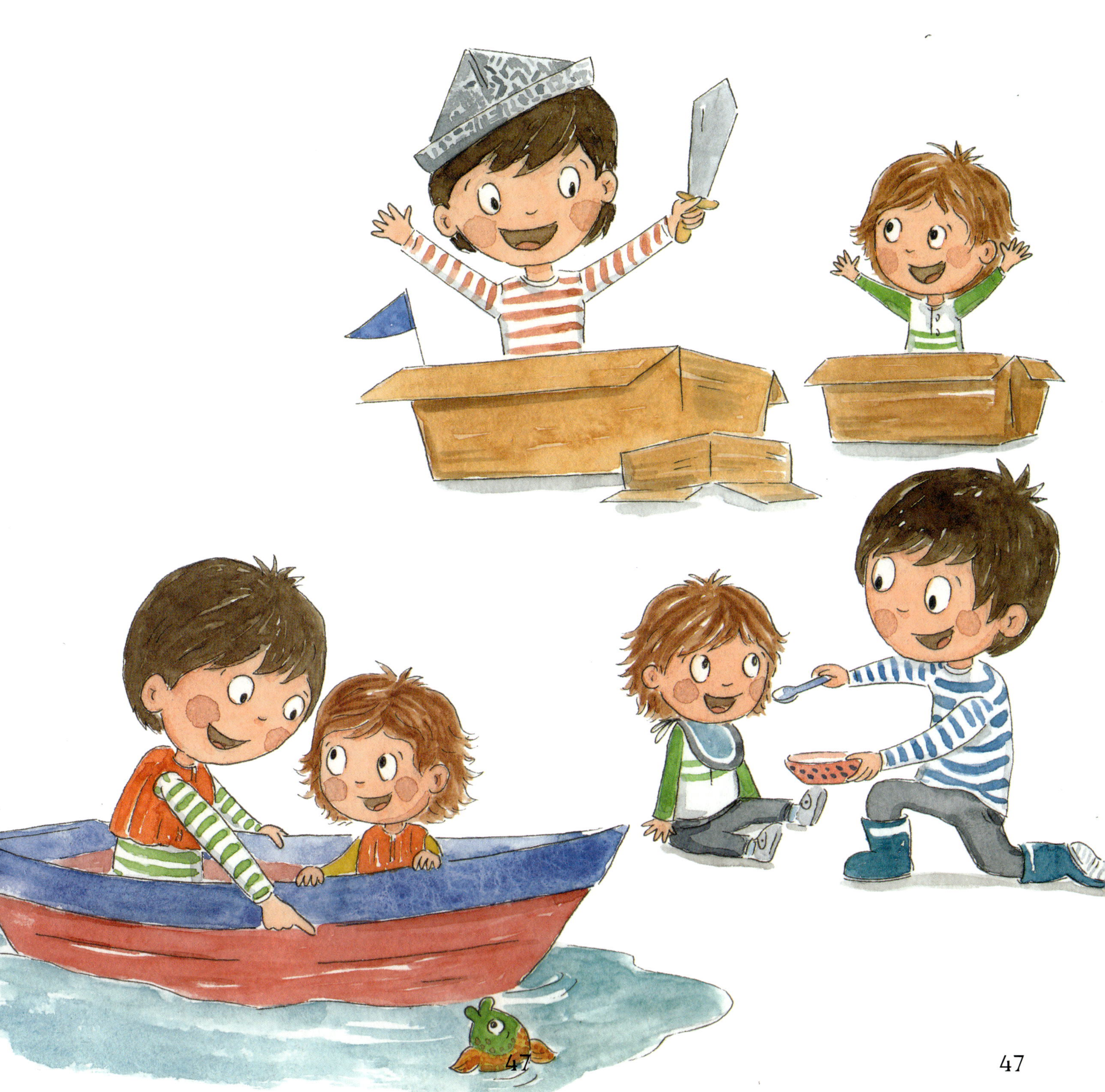